THE IMPORTANCE OF ANIMAL EXPERIMENTATION
FOR SAFETY AND BIOMEDICAL RESEARCH

The Importance of Animal Experimentation for Safety and Biomedical Research

edited by

S. Garattini
Pharmacological Research Institute 'Mario Negri'
Milan
Italy

and

D.W. van Bekkum
Radiobiological Institute 'TNO'
Rijswijk
The Netherlands

Kluwer Academic Publishers
Dordrecht / Boston / London

Library of Congress Cataloging-in-Publication Data

CIP

The Importance of animal experimentation for safety and biomedical research / edited by S. Garattini and D.W. van Bekkum.
p. cm.
Presents the proceedings of an international symposium organized in Stasbourg, Oct. 24-25, 1988.
ISBN-13:978-94-010-7349-3 e-ISBN-13:978-94-009-1904-4
DOI: 10.1007/978-94-009-1904-4
1. Animal experimentation--Congresses. 2. Medicine--Research--Methodology--Congresses. I. Garattini, Silvio. II. Bekkum, D. W. van (Dirk Willem), 1925- .
[DNLM: 1. Animal Welfare--congresses. 2. Animals, Laboratory--congresses. 3. Research--congresses. QY 50 I34 1988]
R853.A53I46 1990
619--dc20
DNLM/DLC
for Library of Congress 89-24434
CIP

Published by Kluwer Academic Publishers,
P.O. Box 17, 3300 AA Dordrecht, The Netherlands.

Kluwer Academic Publishers incorporates the publishing programmes of
D. Reidel, Martinus Nijhoff, Dr W. Junk and MTP Press.

Sold and distributed in the U.S.A. and Canada
by Kluwer Academic Publishers,
101 Philip Drive, Norwell, MA 02061, U.S.A.

In all other countries, sold and distributed
by Kluwer Academic Publishers Group,
P.O. Box 322, 3300 AH Dordrecht, The Netherlands.

printed on acid free paper

Table of Contents

Foreword

Scientists are coming under increasing pressure from activist groups to stop animal experimentation, branded as cruel and unnecessary for improving human health. This attitude, however, stems from an unrealistic evaluation of the situation and distorted information about present scientific knowledge.

There is no question that most medical progress - perhaps all, in fact - has been attained through knowledge derived initially from experiments in various animal species. There is practically no way of replacing animals in these investigations and so-called 'alternative methods' are in reality merely complementary. Tissue cultures, cell, microorganisms, enzymes, membranes, mathematical models - all are useful for preliminary screening tests and for testing hypotheses, but the complexity of a living organism is such that *in vivo* studies are essential before any test can responsibly be made in man.

This book presents the proceedings of an international symposium organized in Strasbourg (October 24-25, 1988), with the aim of assessing present-day requirements as regards animal experimentation in research related to major medical and toxicological problems still awaiting solutions.

Analysis of these chapters will convince any unbiased reader that animals are still needed in the laboratory. However on the positive side scientists are finding ways of using ever-fewer animals as advances are made in technology and non-invasive investigational methods become accessible on a wide scale.

1. The necessity of animal experimentation

SILVIO GARATTINI
Research Institute for Pharmacology 'Mario Negri', Milan, Italy

This volume presents a panorama of biomedical areas in which there is still an urgent need for experimental research. Diseases which affect large numbers of people such as cancer, malaria, leprosy, filariasis, atherosclerosis, dementia, AIDS, as well as rare diseases such as muscular dystrophy, hereditary disorders, inborn metabolic errors and immunodeficiency are all awaiting effective remedies. These calamities call for action. Today the answer is an intensification of biomedical research. It is obvious from the various contributions that progress can only be attained using suitable models of human diseases and these models are based on the use of animals. In no instance is there a single suggestion about using the so-called 'alternative techniques' in place of animals. In this sense it would perhaps be more appropriate to speak of 'complementary' methods because at best they can cut down the number of animals or enable us to obtain more and better information with the same number.

Even in the area of carcinogenesis of chemicals, where the Ames test, with its various modifications, has raised great hopes, there are still no alternative methods to *in vivo* studies. What's more, reports summarizing a large amount of data indicate that the predictive reliability of *in vitro* tests for carcinogenicity is too low since they can still give too many false positive or false negative results.

Historically, models of human diseases reproduced in animals have long been a requisite for discovering new therapies. It is in fact difficult to imagine how to set up *in vitro* techniques for diseases which are expressed under the influence of complex systems such as blood circulation, nervous system regulation, neuroendocrine secretion, immune defences. The animals may not be necessarily the usual ones, as shown by the key role of armadillos in the development of leprosy vaccine and by ferrets in the discovery of antivomiting agents.

Animal research should actually gain fresh impetus from the new technologies available in the area of genetic engineering. The development of transgenic animals is a powerful tool for reproducing human diseases with more accuracy, allowing the expression or the suppression of enzymes, proteins and hormones characteristic of certain human diseases.

S. Garattini (ed.), The Importance of Animal Experimentation for Safety and Biomedical Research, 1–3.

The emphasis on the need for animals is not intended to reduce the importance of *in vitro* techniques; these are particularly useful when a problem has to be studied in simplified well-controlled conditions. There is certainly no need to stress how widely these methods are employed in research laboratories, partly, of course, because they were developed by scientists and not by the opponents of animal experimentation.

Nevertheless, in line with the availability of *in vitro* techniques, the development of better and more sensitive analytical techniques and to the use of appropriate statistical methods, the utilization of animals is decreasing in proportion to the number of scientists. For instance, at the Mario Negri Institute in the last decade the use of laboratory animals has been cut by 40% while in the same period the number of scientists has doubled.

However, pressure from societies for animal protection to orient biomedical research predominantly to *in vitro* studies, and the tendency among biomedical scientists to accept this pressure, may severely jeopardize the outcome of research. It is common knowledge that cells cultured *in vitro* do not retain all their properties and because they are freed from nervous and hormonal influences they acquire some new properties. Therefore to limit research to *in vitro* techniques may be a source of considerable errors and artifacts.

Excessive polarization in discussion of the relevance of *in vitro* techniques is misleading because anyone familiar with biomedical research knows very well that discoveries are just one stage in an unbroken path from clinical observations to laboratory research, from *in vivo* to *in vitro* studies and vice versa, and clinical control of whatever is developed experimentally. The essence of biomedical research lies in this continuous effort and all available techniques – *in vivo* and *in vitro* – must be exploited to reach the goal of improving medical assistance.

The importance of animal research in medicine does not negate the need for regulation to assure humane treatment for animals and to improve the quality of experimental research. In general avoiding suffering, discomfort and stress to animals is in good agreement with the value of results and therefore scientists themselves should be interested in backing these regulations. In this sense the animal protectionists' requests may be useful to the progress of science in the long run if they do not become unrealistic and paralyzing.

A number of regulations can therefore be supported and accepted. They include adequate space and environment for animals; competence of animal caretakers, suitable technicians and scientists, authorizations to institutions, use of anesthesia whenever is an indication. There are however some regulations that scientists cannot accept. These concern essentially the authorization of protocols for experimental research. When working at the frontiers of knowledge it is impossible to decide whether an experiment will be meaningful; history is full of experiments which revealed new information to a particular scientist because he was 'ready' to interpret the results in an unconventional way. Research is like any other human activity and scientists can make mistakes just like other professionals; however, an essential characteristic of research workers is creativity. Only creativity can open up new ideas and new solutions to biomedical problems. But creativity can be judged only *a posteriori*, not *a priori*. It would be absurd to call on a committee, usually including laymen and opponents to the use of animals, to decide whether a given experiment is likely to yield useful results. Advance checks on protocols from anything but the 'legislative' viewpoint are an obstacle to scientific progress and amount to discrimination against science. It has never been suggested that a writer should submit an outline of a future book to be approved by a committee; yet the consequences of a book for society may be more harmful than the sacrifice of a few animals.

Though review of single protocols is unacceptable, checks on the aims of institutions where animals are used for research seem more equitable. Single protocols could be reviewed appropriately inside the institution by *ad hoc* committees, not so much to check the scientific aspects as to verify that all the rules for humane treatment of animals are respected.

Scientists are therefore urged not to agree to preliminary authorization of scientific protocols. The excess of attention for 'animal rights' which seems to be gaining ground in modern society should be viewed critically because it distracts attention from man. If studies on toxicity of xenobiotics are minimized to avoid the use of animals, man will pay because he will certainly be less protected from the chemicals which are part of our life.

The suggestion that we should rely on *in vitro* tests - which are certainly less predictive than extensive *in vivo* tests - undoubtedly has advantages from the point of view of the time and expenses involved. Less time and less cost may appear to be in the interests of industry, but it could amount to potential danger for man. It is indeed impossible to call - as the public does - for better drugs, safer chemicals and a less polluted environment and at the same time to expect the abolition of animal experiments.

This symposium was very useful to verify the present status of research in some fields of medicine and led to the conclusion that today and in the foreseeable future progress in the cure of disease is still linked to the use of animals in research. The proceedings of the symposium will certainly be useful not only for scientists but also as a source of information for divulgation. The symposium, however, has not and will not solve this problem. It is to be expected that antiscientific movements will become more vocal and vigorous in the near future. It is the task and the duty of scientists to explain why we need to use animals and what would be the consequences of banning their use for the progress of medicine. If we are persistent and clear, and particularly if we can resist the temptation to compromise, there is no doubt that rational thinking will prevail.

ETHICAL AND LEGAL ASPECTS

Animal experimentation defended

CARL COHEN
Professor of Philosophy, Medical School, The University of Michigan, Ann Arbor, Michigan, U.S.A.

From my colleagues at the University of Michigan I bring cordial greetings to our friends and hosts in ARTEM and the Istituto di Ricerche Farmacologiche 'Mario Negri', and associated organizations. The intellectual objectives, and the methods of humane inquiry, for researchers on all continents are in essential harmony; I take this opportunity to express satisfaction in our mutual support. My remarks regarding the use of animals as subjects in biomedical experiments are presented under four headings.

Introduction

The battles over the moral wrongs and rights in the use of animals in biomedical research are contested in two distinct philosophical arenas. One of these is utilitarian where the central question is: Does the use of animals as subjects in biomedical research yield a balance of good over evil greater than that yielded by the prohibition of such use? If the answer is yes (as most will conclude), then we will want to ask what restrictions upon the uses of animals in research (if any) will result in the improvement of that balance. Of course the answers to such questions suppose the applicability of some system, call it a calculus, for determining the weights of goods and evils over the short and long term, and the answers assume the fair and rational application of some such system. Precise quantification in the utilitarian weighing will not be possible, obviously, nor is it a requirement for that general moral view to be correct.

The second philosophical arena is deontological and the central question is: Is the moral status of the animals commonly used in research such that, whatever the balance of good and evil flowing from their use it is (or is not) intrinsically wrong to use them as the subjects of medical experiments?

Which of these intellectual courts – the utilitarian or the deontological – is appropriate for the rendering of moral verdicts is a matter upon which, from the time of Socrates, there has been no general agreement. It is certain that we shall not resolve that matter here. The morality of the use of animals

S. Garattini (ed.), The Importance of Animal Experimentation for Safety and Biomedical Research, 7–16.

in research, I submit, may be securely and rightly defended in either of these arenas; but I have not the time here to discuss them both. For an extended treatment of the deontological argument I respectfully call you attention to my earlier essay 'the Case for the Use of Animals in Biomedical Research' [1] appearing in the New England Journal of Medicine on 2 October 1986. Today, especially in the light of the central thrust of this meeting, which is the necessity of animal experiments (for safety and for progress), I think we may most profitably explore the utilitarian arguments over this matter.

Utilitarian principles straightforwardly applied

Criticism of utilitarian moral thinking is widespread among academic philosophers these days; for some, pursuing the attack against utilitarianism may be called a favorite sport. Indeed, it is a moral position that confronts great difficulties, and let me note first, in a grossly oversimple way, why that is so. The principal difficulty with utilitarianism, as a theoretical account of moral judgements, is that it seems often to yield results that are strongly counter-intuitive, and this is true because, in emphasizing the balance of goods over evils, it (allegedly) cannot account for the moral importance of the right distribution of goods and evils. It is not hard to construct a fictional example of an act that we might consider plainly wrong, because outrageously unjust to a given individual - and yet which would provide substantial advantages to so great a number of individuals that we would have little doubt that the balance of utilities favored the act. Now there are ways, within a sophisticated utilitarianism, of fixing that apparent breakdown, by recognizing the additional utility, over the long run, of maintaining certain rules of conduct, so that it becomes not merely the act, but the rule under which the act is done, whose moral status is critical. To this amendment there are rejoinders by the critic, and so on. We are not here to grind all that argument yet finer. Let us suppose, *arguendo*, that we are all utilitarians of one sort or another, or at least that we are close enough to being so that we think it worthwhile to determine, on essentially utilitarian grounds, whether the use of animals in medical research can be morally defined.

When we weigh, as ordinary intelligent people will weigh, the goods and the evils that flow from the use of animals in research, what overall result emerges?

Most of us will conclude that the goods of that use incalculably outweigh the evils. There are evils, surely. Animals (most if not all of them) surely feel pain, and some research entails causing them pain. But most people will think the utilitarian result strongly supports animal use, while earnestly agreeing that we ought to avoid all unnecessary pain or distress to sentient creatures. That will be the conclusion generally reached because, of course, we will put into the balance, as indeed we should, all the benefits for human kind and for animals, that have resulted from research depending essentially upon animal use, and that are likely to depend upon it in the future.

I am not myself a scientist; I do not use animals or do laboratory experiments of any kind. (My direct experience with animals is chiefly limited to the rearing and training of dogs, Briards). One does not need to be himself a scientist, however, to conclude upon review of the evidence that very many great steps in the advance of medicine, and in these days virtually every important step, have been possible only through the use of animal subjects. In recent decades, because effective medical care of humans has become more widely possible, this reliance upon animals as experimental subjects has increased. It would be – as my father used to say – flogging a dead horse to try to list here the truly wonderful things that that use has made possible in the care of human beings, and that would not have been possible if we could not first have experimented upon animals. The point here is not merely that it was through experiments using animals that these advances were achieved, but that only through the use of animals could they have been achieved. Animal use in research has been a necessary condition of much care for human beings that, in retrospect, as in prospect, is precious almost beyond telling.

I cannot forbear flogging that dead horse just a little, for illustrative purposes only. Consider these two medical advances, of very different kind, in which work with animals was, and would always be, irreplaceable.

A) Human hips and other joints are now replaceable by artificial, manufactured joints that make possible mobility for the elderly after injury or deterioration that, for most of human history, has been permanently crippling and an almost sure sign of early death. Not only has the quality of so many thousands of human lives been sustained and improved, but life itself has been advanced. Immobility in the elderly brings on other system failures; we know the dreadful consequences of unrelieved bed rest, even for those in the prime of health. Artificial hips have made possible years of productive life for our parents, our elders and ourselves who would, without such prosthetic devices, soon decline and die. Such devices certainly could not have been developed without extensive experimentation with them on sheep and other animals first. No doubt the sheep did suffer; are there any here who, when sober, would say that the goods done by the advancement of artificial joint replacement are outweighed by the evils of pain caused to the sheep used in their development? That position, and its analog with respect to every other major internal prosthetic device – pacemakers, heart valves, etc. – is the inescapable burden of those who claim that animal research is wrong on utilitarian grounds.

B) Polio, as we know, has now been virtually eradicated for all practical purposes. In my youth – indeed, in my early adulthood – it remained a frightening disease, threatening in every swimming pool, every summer camp, every pace in which boys and girls gathered. It has been virtually eliminated by the use of vaccines whose development was only possible through experimentation upon monkeys; and I think we should face up

> to the fact that many beautiful and endearing monkeys – although not all monkeys are endearing even when they are beautiful, by any means! – were killed in the course of those investigations. Now, please, do the calculations, and answer yourself, as honestly as you can, whether you think, in the interest of the life and comfort of those now dead monkeys, the experimentation that led to the eradication of polio should not have been done. Even if you optimistically believe that one day we will have ways of developing reliable vaccines for deadly diseases other than using live organisms, ask yourself whether the delay in the elimination of polio until that future date would, in retrospect, be defensible on utilitarian grounds. I have no doubt whatever about your answer, if yours is a moral calculus that is truly humane.

Clearly, animals were used in these circumstances not merely as a short-cut, or convenience. We will not permit untried mechanical prostheses being implanted into the innards of human beings – not in my country, not in yours, and I trust, in no country in which a decent respect for the lives of human beings is maintained. Untried vaccines – whose effectiveness can only be tested using animals free of the disease we seek to eliminate – we most assuredly will not introduce into healthy human beings. And are we wrong to protect human beings so? Of course not. We have therefore to choose between the goods accomplished and goods being accomplished, and those to be accomplished, through the use of animals in research, and the good we accomplish (or the evil we avoid) by preserving those sheep and monkeys from the distress imposed upon them in experiment.

Objection and reply

How in the world can an honest utilitarian – a decent, thoughtful person, who truly cares about human well-being, who is not sloppy in analysis, or stupid, or insensitive – how can such a person (say, for illustration, Peter Singer, an Australian philosopher of notable accomplishments, author of Animal Liberation [2]) decide for the sheep at the cost of the humans who will die or suffer in their stead? For Singer does so decide, you know. And he is a very sensitive man, and very, very smart. There are superficial fanatics who speak and write in defense of animals, we know, but he is not one of those. I want to be clear in saying that there are, among my utilitarian critics, many who are certainly not crass or silly. Then what in the world is going through their heads?

We know the answer to that question, because they have told us, at substantial length. In evaluating biomedical experiments using animal subjects they come out with what is (for most of us) a very puzzling result because they give to the life and comfort of the animal – monkey or sheep, dog or rabbit or rat – a value not essentially different from the value they give to the life and comfort of human beings.

This is the key issue in the controversy in this utilitarian arena: *What is the moral status of the experimental animals used in biomedical research and how are we to evaluate the loss of their lives and the distress caused them?* Peter Singer and Ingrid Newkirk, co-chairman of 'People for the Ethical Treatment of Animals' [PETA], the largest organization opposing the use of animals in biomedical research in the United States, ground their arguments upon the same premise: that there is no relevant moral difference between animals (by which I mean the lower animals, of course) and humans. Ms. Newkirk says: '[t]here is no rational basis for saying that a human being has [among all animate beings] special rights. A rat is a pig is a dog is a boy. They're all mammals.' [3]. It is this convinction – shared thinkingly or unthinkingly by so many – that underlies the utilitarian objection to the use of animals.

If you think PETA is not a fair representative of the utilitarian argument, then consider the work of Peter Singer himself, a towering figure in that movement, and who is by his own description explicitly and most assuredly a utilitarian. It is he who has given currency to that ugly neologism in English, 'speciesism', which is the vice, he argues, of giving unjust preference to one species over another. Hence the pains of a rat – no one will doubt that rats feel pain – must be weighed with a tenderness no different from that given to the pains of a human.

I do not know if a synonym has been newly devised. in the French or Italian languages, for 'speciesism'. It is the view that the pain of a sentient creature is simply pain, and all is of essentially the same kind – your pain, the pain of a dog, of a rabbit, of whatever animal you select. The speciesist – of course I am frankly proud of being one – is, on this account, vicious and cruel; the immorality of the speciesist arises; allegedly, from the violation of the principle of equality. Here is the passage in which Singer, in 'Animal Liberation', puts the complaint:

> 'The racist violates the principle of equality by giving greater weight to the interest of members of his own race when there is clash between their interests and the interests of those of another race. The sexist violates the principle of equality by favoring the interests of his own sex. Similarly the speciesist allows the interest of his own species to override the greater interests of members of other species. The pattern is identical in each case.' [2, p. 9].

This argument, I submit, is worse than unsound; it is atrocious. It draws an offensive moral conclusion from a deliberately devised verbal parallelism, in English, that is deceptive and fraudolent. Racism has no rational ground whatever. Differing degrees of respect or concern for humans for no other reason than that they are members of different races is an injustice totally without foundation in the nature of the races themselves. Racists, even if acting on the basis of mistaken factual beliefs, do grave moral wrong precisely because there is no morally relevant distinction between the races. The supposition of such racial differences has led to outright horror. The same is true of the sexes; neither gender is entitled by right to a respect or concern greater than the other. There is no dispute on these matters.

Between species of animate life, however, between (for example) humans on the one hand and cats or rats on the other, the morally relevant differences are enormous, and almost universally appreciated. Humans engage in moral reflection; humans are morally autonomous; humans are members of moral communities, recognizing just claims against their own interest. Human beings have rights - not just rights in law, but moral rights by virtue of their being human, as the Universal Declaration of Human Rights, long defended by the United Nations, expressed with vivid clarity. Humans have a moral status very different from that of cats or rats.

Of course I am a speciesist, as I trust each of you is also. Speciesism is not merely plausible, it is essential for right conduct, because those who will not make the morally relevant distinctions between species are almost certain, in consequences, to misapprehend their true obligations. The weighting they will give to the outcomes of biomedical experiments will be grossly in error.

The analogy between speciesism and racism is therefore not merely unfair to the researcher, it is truly insidious. Every sensitive moral judgment requires that the differing natures of the beings to whom obligations are owed be considered. If all forms of animate life - and is that to include the invertebrate as well as vertebrate? - must be treated equally, and if therefore in evaluating a research program the pains of a rodent count equally with the pains of a human, we are forced to conclude either:

a) that neither humans nor rodents possess moral rights; or

b) that rodents possess all the moral rights that humans do.

Both alternatives are absurd. Yet one or the other must be affirmed if the moral equality of all (vertebrate?) species is to be defended.

Humans owe to other humans a degree of moral regard that cannot be owed to animals. Some humans take on the obligation to support and heal others, humans and animals, as a principal duty in their lives; the fulfillment of that duty may require the sacrifice of very many animals. If biomedical investigators abandon the effective pursuit of their professional objectives because convinced that they may not do to animals what the service of humankind requires, they will fail (on objective, utilitarian grounds) to do their duty. Refusing to recognize the moral differences between species is, I contend, a sure path to calamity.

Rejoinder and response

Critics of animal use are not without some rejoinder. The best of these counterattacks runs as follows: scientific biology permits no sharp line to be drawn between humans and the lower animals; among all the species of animate life there is a continuity that obliges us to weigh the benefits to humans and the evils done to animals on some scale of values essentially the same.

Because of this essential continuity, all animals, even rats and rabbits, cannot be incommensurably inferior to humans. Building upon this foundation, the following argument is presented:
Premise one: In the light of this pervasive continuity, justifying the exploitation of animals on the basis of the benefits it produces would necessarily imply that some human experimental subjects may rightly be exploited in the same way.
Premise two: The exploitation of humans is certainly not morally permissible.
Conclusion: It must therefore be the case that animal use cannot consistently be justified on the basis of the benefits it produces.

This argument has the form of what logicians call *modus tollens* – If P implies Q is true, and Not-Q is true, then not-P must be true. No one will contest the validity of the argument form here; *modus tollens* arguments are certainly valid. If this argument is formally valid, and yet the conclusion is false, one of its premises must be false. Which one? The error is not obscure. The exploitation of human subjects as we exploit animals plainly is not permissible; premise two is surely true. But the first premise is not true. It is not the case that, if the value scales on which the advantages and evils of research are weighed are commensurable for humans and animals, it must then be immoral to treat humans and animals (entities at different points on the scale) differently. No, certainly not. That claim is simply a blunder, and a very misleading one.

In the first place, even if we grant that there is only a single scale for evaluating the evils done to humans and to rats, it would not follow that species falling at very different points on that continuum must be treated similarly. Differences of quantity and relation also matter. Consider this illustration from another context: rich people and poor people, indisputably all moral agents, differ commensurably on a single monetary scale that we all understand full well. Yet we do not think for a moment that this commensurability forbid us to tax the rich as we would not tax the poor. Of course not. Why not? Because important differences may require different moral judgments, even if those differences are along a single scale.

More fundamentally, however, the 'commensurability argument' is built upon a confused and mistaken foundation. The critic points to organic similarities and continuities between humans and other species. No sensible person would deny that there are some such. They do not establish moral commensurability, however. The deeper issue is whether the similarities are of such a kind that what it is plainly immoral to do to humans must also be plainly immoral to do to animals. They are not; overriding the similarities, there are vast differences between species which block our treating them in every matter 'on the same scale'. These differences (even if they prove to have a biological foundation, which is uncertain) are so great, so profound, and so morally relevant that we do say that humans have a moral status of a totally different kind.

Two illustrations of the morally relevant nature of such differences are worth noting here:

1. Of humans we say that we may not experiment upon them without their freely given and fully informed consent. But the moral status of animals is such that, although their bodily organs may be similar, the quest for their consent - informed, voluntary agreement to cooperate in the enterprise - would be a logical absurdity. Humans and rats are profoundly different, and that difference is a consequence of our difference of species.
2. Because humans have a moral status that animals cannot have, we may rightly do to them what they cannot have the right to do to us. We exterminate roaches and rats; sometimes rats eat human babies, and though they have not got the right to do so, they are totally incapable even of conceiving of a moral status for their acts in doing so. Rights are not the kinds of things that rats can be intelligibly said to possess - and it is well to ask oneself why that is so.

Not only do humans have rights that animals cannot have; they can do wrong that animals cannot do. An act is culpable, guilty, when the deed is done with a guilty mind. No rat or sheep can ever commit a crime - although in very primitive societies they were sometimes punished for crimes, as you know - because it is not possible for rats or sheep to have the state of moral awareness necessary for the attribution of wrongfulness to their behavior. Claims of moral wrong and right are simply not applicable to them.

Of course those terms are applicable to us, in our dealings with all creatures who can feel pain. The absence of their rights does not mean that we are free of all obligation to them, of course. Obligations and rights are not reciprocals. Rights entail obligations, yes; but obligations do not necessarily arise from claims of right against us. If my neighbor has a right against me, then I have obligations to respect that right. But I may have other obligations to my neighbor - and to my son, and my students, and even to my dogs - which arise from my relations to them, but not from their rights.

The differences between the species are such that it really does not make sense to say that animals are entitled to the same protection believed essential for humans. If we learn that a lion is killing and eating human children at the forest edge, we hunt it down and kill it, rightly. If we learn that a lion is killing and eating baby zebras in the same region, we do not. Why the difference? Do the baby zebras not feel pain? Do they not fear? Have they not interests? Are they not innocent and endearing? Yes, yes, yes and yes. But they are not endowed with the moral status of the humans we are obliged to protect.

In sum: the critics of animal experimentation who seek to rely upon utilitarian argument consistently fail to draw essential moral distinctions between research subjects having very different moral statuses.

Bring this matter closer to home. Suppose - I trust it did not happen - that as you approached this building by car this morning you accidentally ran over a young squirrel that shot into the path of your vehicle. You are upset and very sorry although you were not at fault. Do you make a big fuss? Do you call the police? An ambulance? Arrange to go to the funeral?

Have a tearful conversation with the parents? See your lawyer? Why not? And why is it right that you do attend to such matters if, God forbid, it were a young human whose body your car had crushed?

There are continuities between squirrels and humans, not to be denied. But the claims that those are moral continuities, and that they prove that all mammals enjoy the same moral status, and are entitled to the same moral regard and protection, is without warrant, and false, and dangerous.

That the refusal to use animals is dangerous is my final point which I can only very briefly outline here. If we are greatly hindered in the use of animals as biomedical subjects, we will be that much more strongly encouraged to use humans in their place. Humans, whose lives and well-being are the proper objects of our duties, are by this restriction likely to be put at serious risk, now and in the future. We are, I trust, going to continue in the development of new surgical procedures, new drugs, new medical therapies of every kind. Whenever we make a step forward we are absolutely compelled, sooner or later, to try what is new for the first time on some living organisms. That will be an experiment. Those experimental subjects will be either animals or humans. At present there is already too much trial with humans before full analysis with animals has been completed. By threatening researchers who use animals, and by harassing them, and by making it difficult and costly for them, we strongly encourage them to move too quickly to dangerous experimentation with humans. This we certainly ought not do.

There is one other alternative: to slow the course of medical advance. This, also, we must not do. The choices for biomedical investigators come down to these three:

1. Use humans extensively in biomedical experimentation that must result in their injury and death; or
2. Use animals – chiefly rats and mice, but also dogs and rabbits and primates and other species – in such biomedical experimentation; or
3. Do neither, by ceasing to do such experiments.

The first of these alternatives is morally out of the question. If the third is also a violation of our moral duties – as the papers presented in this special Congress, illustrating the essential role of animal experimentation for safety and for medical advances of the most precious kind, make vividly clear – then it follows inexorably that the biomedical use of animals is not merely permissible, but is morally obligatory. That is why I contend that systematic opposition to the use of animals in biomedical research is dangerous to humans over the short and long term, and is inhumane, and is the result of a series of unfortunate errors in moral reasoning.

References

1. Cohen C (1986) 'The case for the use of animals in biomedical research', *The New England*

Journal of Medicine 315: pp. 865–870
2. Singer P (1975) *Animal Liberation*, Avon Books, New York
3. McCabe K (Aug 1986)'Who will live, who will die?', *The Washingtonian Magazine*

The ethics of animal use in biomedicine

T.L.S. SPRIGGE
Philosophy Department, David Hume Tumor, University of Edinburgh, U.K.

I hope that the time is past when those who use animals for scientific purposes regard criticisms from animal welfare and animal rights movements as the mere sentimental effusions of people with more heart than head and with a basically anti-scientific frame of mind. The leading figures of these movements have for some time past been people of some academic distinction while the movement for the replacement of animals in biomedical research and testing is spear-headed in Britain by FRAME (Fund for the Replacement of Animals in Medical Experiments) periodical, ATLA (Alternatives to Laboratory Animals), publishes work of high scientific quality. Criticisms of animal experimentation from such sources cannot be laughed off and I hope that this conference will give some attention to them.[1] It is desirable that both practitioners and critics of animal experimentation should be prepared to learn from each other and not necessarily think of all those on the other side as either villains or sentimentalists.

This conference is concerned with the alleged necessity of animal experimentation for biomedical science. In this address I shall offer you some classification of the positions which philosophers and other moral thinkers have taken to the use of animals for scientific purposes, with some brief indication of my own view. For purposes of this paper I shall mean by an animal 'any member of the five *vertebrate* classes, i.e. non-human mammals, birds, reptiles, amphibians and fish'.[2]

Some think that a philosopher has little to contribute in this area, for to some philosophy seems remote from the practical realities of the world. To this I shall say that moral philosophy is only a particularly systematic attempt to think out the foundations of ethics and their implications for desirable practice, and that to be against moral philosophy is to be against the use of reason in coming to ethical conclusions.

But some may think that most philosophers (or at least philosophers without a scientific training) who criticise the use of animals in science are to be condemned along with animal welfare-ists in general for taking up positions on matters they do not understand. In reply to this I might say that this principle would make it inappropriate for anyone to condemn slavery if they

S. Garattini (ed.), The Importance of Animal Experimentation for Safety and Biomedical Research, 17–28.

have not lived in a slave state, or apartheid if they have not lived in a racialist state. Ethics is surely everyone's business. It is obvious that those engaged in research using animals are going to be better informed on the subject than most of those who are not, but that does not invalidate the critics' moral concern or discredit their serious efforts and some degree of success in getting hold of relevant facts. And if critics of animal experimentation are accused of appealing to emotion rather than reason there is no shortage of grounds for this charge on the other side.[3]

I believe that anyone who looks into the matter seriously will, if he thinks that the sufferings of animals matter at all, find it hard not to conclude that much research has gone on in respectable institutions which is beyond the pale.[4] If such a person wishes to clarify the moral issues to himself it may be helpful to consider which of the following five main moral views on animal experimentation seems the most satisfactory basis for evaluating particular cases.

The *first* view, which might be called pure humanism, is the view that *there are no moral restrictions at all on what humans have a right to do to animals in pursuit of their own goals.* Sometimes this is supported on the basis of the view that animals really do not feel pain, or perhaps are not genuinely sentient at all. (The seventeenth century rationalist philosopher, Descartes, himself a vivisectionist, held this view. In our own day the psychologist Nick Humphreys denies consciousness or sentience to most animals, even most mammals.)

The *second*, only slightly less extreme, view is that animals, even though capable of genuine suffering, are nonetheless so lacking in all the features which mark our fellow humans as proper objects of our moral concern that *their interests should always take second place to those of humans.* That is, where it makes no difference to humans whether research is done one way or another we should try to obviate suffering for animals, but we should never let the suffering of animals deter us from doing what in other respects represents the most efficient way in which we can pursue the good of humans.

The special distinction of humans is usually thought of as being their rationality and, closely related to this, their linguistic powers. Supporters of the second view sometimes see this as a reason for saying that *humans* have moral rights but that it would be nonsensical to ascribe similar rights to animals. For rights, so it is argued, can only pertain to those who can grasp the fact that they possess them and thus can press or perhaps waive them. (On the face of it, this disallows rights to babies and badly retarded humans.)

The *third and fourth* views both rely on the ethical position known as utilitarianism. According to this *actions are justified only if they increase the general balance of happiness over unhappiness in all sentient creatures.*

The *third* view is that this utilitarian principle justifies extensive use of animals for research, some of which involves pain for them, because the benefit to human, and perhaps animal, health achieved outweighs the suffering for the animals. It follows that it would be justifiable to do experiments of a painful sort either on humans or animals if the good to be achieved (in terms of further suffering prevented) outweighed this. However, it is held that to use humans as involuntary experimental subjects would be objectionable because human life would be wretched in a situation where everyone lived in fear that they themselves might be used in this way. Therefore experimentation must be confined to animals, for they will only suffer the immediate pain, and there will be no general panic among the relevant species of animals at large.

The *fourth* view is again utilitarian. What matters, it says, is the maximisation of welfare generally. However, utilitarians of this fourth type claim that, at least as things stand, there is a vast amount of (often repetitive) animal experimentation the good achieved by which does not outweigh the immense amount of suffering it causes and the blunting of the moral sensitivities of those involved in it – whose result is likely to be further, less justified painful experimentation. It is argued that once we begin to tolerate the infliction of suffering on helpless creatures in our hands, we will never manage to restrict this to those cases where it really is for the general good, including the good of animals.

The *fifth* view says that *each individual human or animal has certain basic moral rights in virtue of which she cannot be legitimately used to advance the welfare of others, without his/her consent.* So even if the greatest happiness of the greatest number, taking both animals and humans into account, would be advanced by actions involving suffering for some particular animal, say one used in a medical experiment, it is wrong thus to exploit one creature for the benefit of others. (The fact that this may in a certain sense be done in the wild is not to the point, for we have to consider what moral agents, who can think about the matter, have the right to do, not what may inevitably happen in nature.)

Of course, when moralists speak of rights in this context they are speaking of moral, not of legal, rights. It is assumed that individuals can have moral rights whether or not the law has acknowledged these rights and thus made them into legal rights. By 'rights' I shall mean 'moral' rather than 'legal rights' throughout this talk.

I do not understand how any decent and intelligent person can support the first of the five views I listed. I suspect that the thesis that animals are not conscious can only be sustained through confusion between consciousness and self-consciousness. This latter term is susceptible of various shades of meaning. It is by no means obvious that most mammals lack *self-consciousness* in all important senses of the phrase. Anyway that would not prevent their being *conscious*, in the sense of having genuine perceptual experience and feelings of pleasure, pain and of various emotions.

The second view implies that there is such a vast divide between humans and animals that what happens to an animal never really matters in anything like the way what happens to a human does. Well, obviously there are great differences, but to think them so great that animal suffering does not matter in essentially the same way as human suffering does has little reason to it and surely shows lack of imaginative insight.

Leaving views three and four aside for the moment, let me say a word about the fifth view. This depends heavily upon the notion of a moral right. What is a moral right? Some maintain that it makes no sense to ascribe rights to individuals to whom duties cannot be ascribed. But this means that rights cannot be ascribed to human babies and perhaps people suffering from certain forms of mental disability, and few would go along with this.

When we discuss whether animals have rights or not, it is important to distinguish between two grounds on which it may be denied that they do.

(1) The first ground turns on the wholesale rejection of the notion of a moral right. It declares it a merely rhetorical expression which adds nothing to the essentials of judgement about what it is right or wrong to do to those said to have the right and is useless in the solution of moral questions.

However, so long as one holds any moral views at all about the permissible treatment of people it is difficult to avoid using the term 'rights' in their expression. It may be replied that once one has said that it is very wrong to treat fellow human beings in various ways, say by torturing them to extract information, affirming their right not to be treated thus adds nothing and gives no extra ground for condemning it. I reply that it does add something, for it highlights the fact that there is something about people, namely their capacity to suffer, that makes it wrong to treat them in this way. Thus the word 'right' directs attention to the status of the person who has the right as no other word can do. And the question stands how far animals have a similar status;

(2) The second ground for denying rights to animals registers a wish to distinguish the grounds for moral judgements about permissible behaviour to our fellow humans and to animals. While the wrongness of torturing a human can properly be expressed by reference to his rights, it can play no proper part (it says) in expressing any view about what it is permissible or not to do to animals.

Such a restriction upon the use of the word 'rights' is unfortunate, for it suggests that the reason why it is wrong to ill-treat animals is radically different from the reason why it is wrong to ill-treat humans, and that, I believe, is a mistake. For the reason is the same in each case, namely that any reasonable sense of what it must be like from the victim's own point of view, whether it be a human or an animal, to be subjected to certain sorts of treatment, will or would produce moral revulsion and consequent condemnation on the part of any adequately sensitive person.

In the light of this I suggest that the best way of using the term 'right' is so that an individual can be said to have a moral right to something when there are grounds for complaint on his behalf if he does not have it, serious grounds for complaint, that is, against rational agents who are (at least partly) to be blamed for his not having it. Used in that way, we can say that babies have rights as much as adults, even though they have no duties and cannot themselves press their rights. And once one uses 'rights' in this sense one can only deny that animals have rights if one means that there is never ground for complaints being registered on their behalf. To acknowledge that animals have rights in this sense is to acknowledge that what happens to them matters in the same essential way as it matters what happens to humans, namely that they are conscious creatures whose lives can be more or less enjoyable, or more or less wretched, from their own subjective point of view, of which anyone of appropriate sensitivity will feel the need to take some account. So I certainly do think that both humans and animals have moral rights in this sense.

To say that animals have rights in this sense is to leave it open precisely what their rights are. These can hardly extend to the whole gamut of human rights, for example, they will not include the right to free speech in anything very like the usual sense. And to allow that all animals have some rights is not necessarily to lump them all together and say that the rights of an ape are to be equated with the rights of a fish.

Still, I agree with utilitarian philosophers who say that appeal to a moral right is more a way of reporting a moral conclusion than a way of justifying it. The first and most obvious reason why the use of torture is wrong is the terrible nature of the experience for the victim. A second reason is the immense value for human life of retaining or developing forms of fellow feeling and compassion incompatible with involvement in the infliction of it. This is so important that even if there are rare cases where the importance of the end might otherwise seem to outweigh the victim's sufferings, the use of torture should still be disallowed on the ground that its use on one occasion will break down a sentiment against its use of longer term value to humanity than any immediate goal. On these grounds I am prepared to insist that it is always wrong to torture a human being, and I think it quite appropriate and rhetorically helpful to express this by saying that humans have a right not to be tortured. But this does not so much give the reason why it is wrong to torture people as express this wrongness emphatically. So I do not think that an appeal to animal rights such as is made by the fifth point of view I mentioned deals with the issue at the most basic level. The only serious alternative seems to be some version of the utilitarian principle – and the version I would favour implies that one should never inflict suffering except in the interests of preventing worse suffering which is certainly or almost certainly only avoidable by doing so.[5]

That leaves the third and fourth views and it is the fourth which I support. Surely an immense amount of testing and experimentation goes on which cannot possibly be justified as achieving a good which outweighs the harm done.[6] I suggest also that much should be stopped, even of what seems of enormous utility, because it is part of a general system in which sentiments of concern for forms of sentient life which cannot protect themselves from human exploitation are suppressed or not allowed to develop. Surely the preservation of our own reluctance to inflict suffering on innocent creatures is itself a great good, to be put in the balance when we consider how much suffering it is justifiable to inflict on animals even for research likely to be of real benefit to men (and perhaps animals). Certainly those who work for the discovery of cures for disease are by and large actuated by humane sentiment, and I do not insist here that absolutely all use of animals for medical experimentation is wrong. However, unless there is something more than a merely token acknowledgement of the bad side of it (as when it is called a necessary evil), I think there will be a lack of real effort to find alternatives. It is only when we take seriously the immensely bad thing which it is for animals to suffer and to be unable to live the kinds of lives they can enjoy, and the way in which human nature is depraved by the suppression of humane sentiment, that there will be any really serious attempt to reduce it, I can only see this attempt becoming really serious if it is agreed (1) that humans must move towards a total ban on painful experiments at some date in the not too distant future (a decision which would give enormous impetus to the development of alternatives) and (2) that until then, maximal concern is given to ensuring laboratory animals a decent life.

I would express this view by saying that animals have a strong *prima facie* right not to be subjected to pain for human purposes, and that this, if it can be over-ridden at all, can only be over-ridden in cases of peculiar crisis, and where there is a continuing effort to move towards methods which do not involve suffering. Although I do not put such weight on the notion of a right as the fifth view, I do think that we need to talk of rights here if we are to put the kind of serious warning post in the way of the ready use of animals for experimentation which any genuine recognition of the fact that their suffering is as real as is ours will make us find appropriate. At the very least anyone doing research with animals must continually ask himself how far his work is compatible with this recognition.

I have said nothing about painless killing. No one who eats meat can think that killing of animals is normally wrong. That objection does not come home to me very seriously personally as I am a vegetarian. One reason for this is that I think that in the interests both of animals and of humans, if the kinds of compassionate sentiments to life at large which are needed for the future welfare even of the human race are to be adequately cherished, we should move as far as we can to a non-killing society. However, killing animals is much less bad than causing serious or prolonged suffering. Quite apart from causing obvious pain we should avoid imposing on animals the kind of distresses which, I believe, must be associated with inability to live the kind of life to which evolution has adapted them. Thus keeping animals in conditions which frustrate their inherited behaviour patterns, killing them, and causing them pain are all serious evils, both in terms of what it does to the animals and what it does to us. It is not enough to say that we should avoid this as much as possible, for what does 'possible' mean? We should acknowledge that the welfare of animals should sometimes outweigh our own, since their feelings are as genuine as ours. We should be particularly concerned to avoid ways of treating them which encourage us to think of them as mere physical raw material for us to use in whatever way is convenient for us.

That leaves many questions open, but I suggest that if we clearly recognize that animals are individual conscious subjects in the same sense as we are, a preparedness to rely for ever on experiments involving pain, or frustrating restraints, as a permanent backup to human welfare will seem increasingly repellent, and that the search for a life style no longer dependent upon massive animal suffering will become more and more essential for our own human peace of mind.

What can be deduced by way of more concrete recommendation from the ethical position I have outlined? The use of animals in a scientific context are of various types[7] including:

1. basic research;
2. extraction of products, e.g. antisera;
3. discovery of drugs, pesticides;
4. toxicity testing;
5. education and training.

So far as the ethics of the matter goes, such procedures can be divided into four main categories.

A) Those which involve distress or pain for the animals as an unavoidable aspect of the procedure in question.

B) Those which involve killing of animals but which do not necessarily involve suffering.

C) Those which do not involve distress or pain for the animals except in the most minimal degree and do not involve killing of the animals as part of the procedure. This category includes behavioural studies which are either of a purely observational kind or which include some interferences with the animal's environment in order to study its consequent behaviour but where the disturbance is hardly of a sort to cause any real distress.

Everyone will probably agree that these three categories of procedure are of decreasing moral questionability. (A) and perhaps (B) are the more questionable ones, and the most obvious considerations bearing on their justifiability are:

1. Purpose of the procedure
2. Possibility of achieving the same purpose without use of animals
3. Effort used to avoid duplicating work already done.

Actual carrying out of procedure of each kind may be classified according as to how much more suffering they in practice involve than the nature and purpose of the procedure requires. There seem to be four main heads here: (1) how much, if any, distress of a kind not essential to the procedure the animal actually undergoes in the course of it, (2) how far the animal is kept for the whole of its life in conditions allowing it a decent life, (3) the eventual fate of the animal when use of it has finished, in those cases where the procedure does not, of itself, involve the animal's death, (4) how far an essentially comparable procedure could have been carried out on another species which it is reasonable to think would suffer less in the process.

Type A procedures, which involve distress or pain for the animals as an unavoidable aspect of the procedure in question, are the only ones I can deal with here, for brevity's sake and I shall concentrate on the use of animals in research.

The first thing to realize is that they are certainly *prima facie* wrong and that the burden of proof is on the person who supports them. For suffering is the very paradigm of evil and its infliction must be wrong unless the badness of the suffering is definitely outweighed by the good it does.

What form may this good take? I suggest that it can only legitimately take the form of the prevention of more suffering. The main alternative is the promotion of new forms of positive satisfaction. But it is a very dubious morality that justifies causing suffering in one group of creatures merely in order to add to the pleasures of life for another group. For apart from anything else humans – and it is virtually always the happiness of human beings that is in question – are capable of a diversity of forms of happiness and it is surely for the general welfare that we should learn to enjoy ourselves in ways not deriving from the suffering of others. So I suggest that any infliction of suffering on animals in order to add to human happiness, rather than to reduce human misery, is out. That seems to rule out, among other things, causing suffering to animals in the course of field sports and trapping them for luxurious furs.

It is arguable that from the same point of view the causing of suffering in the interests of the extension of pure knowledge, where this is not done for the sake of relief from suffering, should not be allowed. There would appear to be just three main reasons why knowledge is good: (1) because its acquisition and possession is a main human satisfaction; (2) because it adds indirectly to the means of positive happiness; (3) because it can be used for the relief of suffering. But (1) and (2) are ruled out by the principle that one should not inflict suffering merely in order to promote human happiness.

It follows that the only possible justification for inflicting suffering on animals is as a means to the relief of human and perhaps animal suffering. Now it will be said in defence of painful experimentation that it is advancing knowledge essential for the attack upon disease, physical and mental, or for the treatment of injuries. However such a justification cannot be valid unless:

1. The probability of the result is evidently greater than the probability that, if use of this means were prohibited, the same end would not be gained by another means.
2. The general weakening of humane sentiments in a community which allows such practices is not a greater evil than the evil which is to be removed.

I do not say that it is often easy to decide whether either of these propositions are true, but where there is not excellent reason for thinking that they are, it seems evident that we should avoid the certain evil of inflicting the suffering.

And this is particularly the case where what is in question is research directed at the increase of general scientific knowledge with only a vague promise of results for the treatment of disease which could not be gained elsewhere. In this connection I recommend consideration of the contention of Andrew Rowan that the extent to which biomedical research is most helpful in finding cures for diseases when it is not directed specifically at such an end is very dubious.[8] One should also ponder the claim of Mary Midgley that where knowledge of very fundamental facts about life is in question there is always going to be more than one means of finding them out.[9]

But that leaves us with cases here there really is good reason to think that a research programme will rescue humanity from the scourge of some appalling disease or for the palliation of the effects of some disaster.[10] If the suffering to be relieved is much greater than that inflicted on animals there are some difficulties in a utilitarian objecting to it. Yet there is one consideration which may still give ground for pause and which is surprisingly neglected. The resources-financial and human-devoted to projects involving animal suffering are always going to be resources which could be directed elsewhere. Since humanity has so many ills, not only in the form of disease but in the form of famine, war, and so forth it is a serious question where the energies directed at conquering diseases through painful research of various kinds would go if such research were prevented. If those scientists whose work involves painful experimentation on animals really are motivated primarily by a concern for human welfare their talents and those of their potential successors could surely be put to other equally beneficial work – indeed there is plenty of room simply for the better application even of existing knowledge. For if the end is the improvement of the quality of sentient life in general, in particular the reduction of suffering, and if resources are limited, priority should be given to activities calculated to relieve suffering other than by way of causing it.

From this consideration I extract the following principle: Painful experimentation can only be justified when it is overwhelmingly probable that it will lead to a reduction of suffering greater than that which it causes and greater than could be brought about by any activities competing with that research for limited resources in terms of finance and man power. I would supplement this principle by saying that the general desirability of promoting humane attitudes to sentient life at large should serve as extra weighting on the negative side whenever the acceptability of painful research is being considered.

An outsider may suspect that if all painful experimentation were prohibited an enormous fillip to other forms of research would be given so that alternative procedures would be found where at present it is denied that they are possible.

All this gives some support to the view that painful experimentation should be prohibited. At the very least it suggests that the case in its defence needs to be much stronger than it has been.

That stronger defence, to be convincing must not take the form of depicting animal welfare-ists as anti-scientific sentimentalists, but must come rather from recognizing the rightness of at least a very great deal of their case. Defence of painful experimentation cannot be taken seriously unless (1) it comes from people who roundly condemn a great deal of what has gone on in laboratories with the same degree of outrage as anti-vivisectionists show; (2) the experimenters show a real sense that the infliction of suffering on animals is something extremely undesirable in itself and only ultimately to be justified in a limited number of cases of a kind they are doing everything possible to make unnecessary by the development of alternatives; (3) the conditions in which the animals are bred (or captured) do not involve distress of any removable kind; (4) it is not thought a waste of resources to spend a considerable amount on improving the animals' living conditions so that they can actually get some 'satisfaction' out of their lives, and (5) that the research is genuinely directed at the alleviation of very serious evils worse than any others from which they may be diverting resources.

All this has concerned the morality of painful experiments, but a word is in order about the killing of animals.

Consider first why killing *humans* is for the most part, wrong? I suggest that it is the ultimate act of aggression and expresses the view that the other person does not matter in his own right. A society or world in which people are ready to kill each other for their own advantage is one in which there is little respect for the way in which the other person's life is important to him in just the way that one's own is for oneself. Essentially the same applies to the killing of animals. It is an act of aggression against them. That surely gives a reason for wishing for a society in which people have a strong resistance to killing animals.

But while I think animal suffering can be as, or almost as, bad a thing as human suffering I do not think the same is true of animal death.

First there is the point that social arrangements which would allow one human to be killed for the sake of others would lead to widespread misery and dread, on the part of the likely victims in expectation, and the victim's loved ones after the event, whereas this is much less the case with animals. Therefore it is much more easy to justify the killing of animals for the sake of using their organs in *in vitro* testing and research. At any rate it would be such an extraordinary advance in the human treatment of animals if painful experimentation were abandoned that I think one can leave the matter of killing aside as a much less urgent issue. But that does not mean there should not be a serious attempt to reduce the number of animals killed for the benefit of man. And certainly there is every reason to insist that animals who are destined to be killed for the benefit of man should be given a really good life till they meet their fate.

I do not think that the use of animals in the testing or production of products raises substantially different questions though in some cases it is perhaps harder to form a reasonable view. Where this involves suffering one cannot justify it unless it is an indispensable means to an overridingly desirable goal (and where pursuit of that goal is not an alternative to the pursuit of another equally desirable goal which does not involve suffering). This condition will only be satisfied where it is genuinely impossible to find other means of testing or producing the product and where the product is absolutely essential for the relief of serious misery. It is not enough that it merely adds something positive to human welfare. Nor is it enough that any alternatives are more expensive where this excuse is offered by anyone failing to agitate for resources for the alternative.

Thus in the case of much routine toxicological testing of products to be marketed in competition with existing products which really serve the purpose well enough the consideration that it lowers the whole readiness to respect sentient life in all its forms should be decisive against it, without the need for minute weighing-up of benefits and harms. We are not sensitive people if we are happy to see what are essentially consumer goods improved in fundamentally unimportant ways at the cost of massive animal suffering, and part of man's progress to a better attitude to other creatures must be through the refusal to use such products.

There are many ethical aspects of this complicated question on which I do not have space to say much. One important matter concerns the degree of right different species have. If it is worse to hurt or kill a human than to hurt or kill an ape, is it worse to hurt or kill an ape than a fish or even a rat? Every creature which is sentient at all (that is, which can either enjoy life or suffer) is properly regarded as an end in itself in the sense that it matters what happens to it, not just on account of the effects on other individuals, but on account of what it is like for that creature to live through that experience. The really big divide is between those who think of animals as so inferior in moral status to humans that they are there simply to be used by us as we find convenient and those who think that the quality of an animal's life matters in the same intrinsic way as that of a human does, though possibly less. If all parties to the dispute over animal experimentation could agree to the second proposition it would become much easier for the matter to be debated with mutual respect.

Notes

1. Among important critical works by philosophers are the seminal *Animal Liberation* (London, 1976) by the Australian philosopher, Peter Singer, *The Case for Animal Rights* (London, 1983) by the American philosopher Tom Regan, and *The Moral Status of Animals* (Oxford, 1977) by Stephen Clark, *Animal Rights and Human Morality* by Bernard Rollin and *Animals and Why They Matter* by Mary Midgley (London, 1983) and Peter Singer again in chaps 3–5 of his *Practical Ethics* (Cambridge, 1979).

   These are serious works, not at all sentimental, which claim that there is a real failure of moral insight in those who carry out and support much standard animal experimentation. The most serious rejoinder of which I know is *Man and Mouse* (Oxford, 1984) by the pharmacologist William Paton, and there is also a work by the philosopher, R G Frey, called *Interests and Rights; The Case against Animals* (Oxford, 1980). A particularly important work is the highly informative *Of Mice, Models and Men; A Critical Evaluation of Animal Research* by Andrew Rowan, (State University of New York Press, Albany, 1984) which takes a middle position.

2. This was the definition of 'animal' used in the recent *US Congress Office of Technology Report on Alternatives to Animal Use* see summary in ATLA 14, p. 291. How far animal welfare-ists' concern should extend to other forms of animal life, such as insects, is a problem I must set aside.
3. *Of Mice, Models and Men* by Andrew N. Rowan, Albany, New York, Chapter 3, contains an interesting account of the quality of debate on both sides.
4. I will not cite examples here beyond remarking on one extreme case which received a good deal of publicity recently in my local press in Scotland, that of experiments on brain damage carried out on baboons and other primates at the University of Pennsylvania, brains from which were received for research by the medical faculty at Glasgow as a result of which the matter received some publicity in the Scottish press.

   There was a report of this in *The Scotsman* for November 16, 1984. For further details on the research at Pennsylvania see the *Annual Pictorial Review 1985* of the Scottish Society for the Prevention of Vivisection.
5. Some qualifications may be necessary to this principle but they are not ones which affect the present issue.
6. If a product can only safely be put on the market after testing on animals, and does not represent any very serious advance on existing products which there is good reason to think safe, then anyone who is not against introduction of the new product cannot be said to take animal welfare very seriously. That the existing products were tested on animals does not in any way affect this point. But surely one may also say that there are types of product tested by toxicologists which the human race could have been quite without it being clear that life would have therefore been much worse; this is particularly obvious, it might be thought, in the case of many cosmetic products. Would it not have been better to do without these commodities and retain our humane sentiments?
7. Derived from Rowan, *op. cit.* p. 10–15 and from personal communication by Michael Balls.
8. Andrew Rowan: *Of Mice, Models and Men*, p. 17.
9. Mary Midgley: 'Why Knowledge Matters' in *Animals in Research*, ed. D. Sperlinger, pp. 319–336, Chichester, J. Wiley and Sons.
10. Ideally a word about defence research should be said at this point. Insofar as that is part of the defence programme it raises the whole question of how far that is ethical. But even if it is ethical, which many of us may doubt, all the cautions about the use of animals for research aimed at more strictly medical groups apply at least as strongly. Where it is not so much part of the defence programme but directed simply at reducing the suffering and death caused in war it raises much the same issues as other biomedical research.

Legal and political problems of animal experimentation the 'Swiss battle'

FRANK BRIDEL
Pharma Information, Basel, Switzerland

The word vivisection dates back to the 18th century, and at the time it was coined it made sense. The bulk of animal trials were of a surgical nature and, since anaesthesia had not yet been discovered, any intervention of this kind, either on humans or on animals, was extremely painful.

As feelings of sympathy grew – fortunately – during the 19th century, antivivisectionism was born, spread, and kept its name even after the introduction of anaesthesia. Nowadays, many adversaries of animals trials still call themselves antivivisectionists, despite two radical changes in the laboratories. Firstly, animal trials centre much more on pharmacology and toxicology than on surgery. Secondly, surgery is always performed under anaesthesia. In fact, the word vivisection is a double anachronism. It is unfortunately still used, above all by those interested in dramatizing the situation, because of its cruel connotations, at least in language areas where the etymology or origin of this word is more or less transparent.

Anyhow, hostility to experimentation on animals is still with us and in the last 5–10 years has reached a new peak. The result of this was, for a while, direct threats against scientists, even terrorist attack, mainly in the United Kingdom. And, in parallel or as an alternative to this sort of action, pressure was brought to bear on governments and parliaments to enforce more stringent legislations.

This led to the recent political battles in the UK and in Germany to obtain new laws which, in the end, seemed acceptable to scientists. But still there is a movement trying to make these laws, or their enforcement more severe. In the United States, mostly at individual state level, there is permanent agitation towards this end.

But there is only one country in which, by virtue of its institutions of direct democracy, citizens recently had to vote for or against animal trials and many will have to do so again in a few years. I will, from now on, concentrate on the Swiss campaign scientists from the universities and the industry had to organize in order to avoid what was tantamount to forbidding animal trials in a small country, but a country strongly dedicated to biological research.

Before I speak of the campaign, some explanation of the very complicated

S. Garattini (ed.), The Importance of Animal Experimentation for Safety and Biomedical Research, 29–34.

Swiss system of direct democracy is called for. I shall concentrate on what is indispensable to understand what happened in the campaign, by sketching out the following points: if 100.000 citizens put their signature to a proposal for amendment of the Federal Constitution, it is compulsory that, within a defined period, all the citizens be called upon to express their opinion in a vote. This will happen only after a debate, first within the Government, then in Parliament (both houses). After that both Government and Parliament will tell the citizens whether they recommend a vote of yes or no. The final decision will rest nevertheless with the people who go and vote.

Now, let us come to the recent story. In 1981, a new law on animal protection was brought into force in Switzerland. This law contains new rules on animal trials. They are considered to be the most severe in the world, but the law's severity was considered insufficient by the most passionate antivivisectionists, and they launched a proposal of amending the Federal Constitution by introducing a new paragraph completely prohibiting animal trials. And they got the 100.000 signatures they needed, so that from that moment the whole procedure I have just described.

Of course, scientists and also many other professionals, fortunately, were immediately convinced that acceptance of the proposal would simply kill biological research in that very country where you probably find the highest concentration of this activity in relation to the small population of six million inhabitants.

Starting in 1983, a campaign was organized, with competent people and, fortunately, the broad support of all the professions interested in research and health, such as universities and other research institutes, the research-based pharmaceutical industry, physicians, pharmacists, veterinarians and chemists. Moreover, since the problem had serious political and economic implications, all 26 member states of the Confederation (the so-called cantons) were against the amendment, as were all the political parties with the exception of the communists, the extreme left and the Swiss 'green' party. Conscious of the risks for jobs within research and related activities, the trade unions were also against the proposed amendment, as well as, last but not least, the national Society for the Protection of Animals.

Of course, I am simplifying, because all these organizations did not have such clearcut opinions right from the beginning. A lengthy process of information and motivation was needed to achieve this, but it did so quite easily. The same can be said of Government and Parliament, with the result that they both recommended that the citizens should reject the amendment. One of the two chambers even voted this recommendation unanimously. In a second phase, the battle overcome had to be fought to convince the final decision makers, that is the citizens, who often vote against the official recommendations by Government or by Parliament.

What we did first and, at shorter and shorter intervals, during the campaign, was opinion polls. This is of capital importance, because you cannot run a campaign without knowing what the people think.

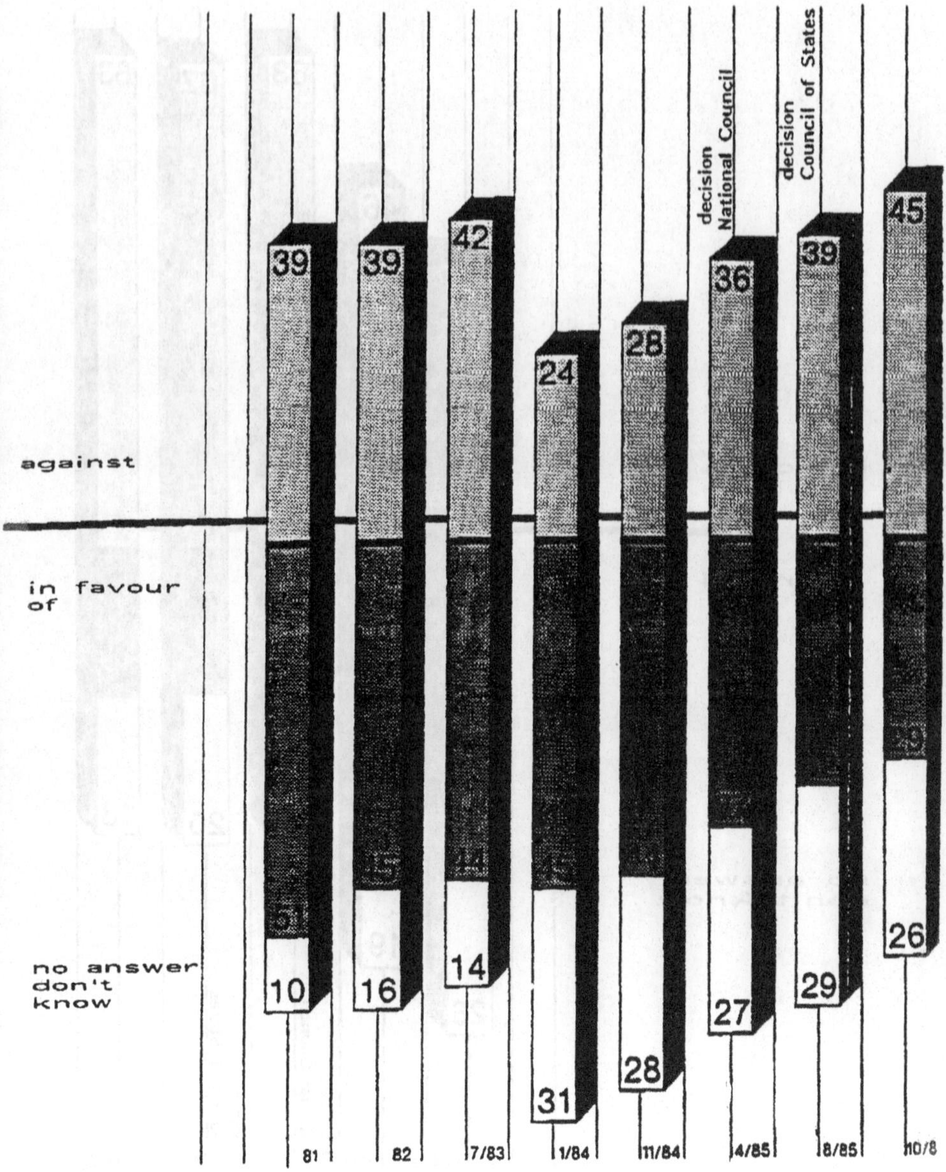

Fig. 1. Direct question. How are you going to vote, in favour or against the initiative (abolishment of animal trials)?

As Figures 1 and 2 show, we always put two questions: first, 'How are you going to vote?' and second, 'How do you think the majority will vote?' Experience tells that normally, the final result is in between. The situation at the onset was not encouraging at all, and something happened that one

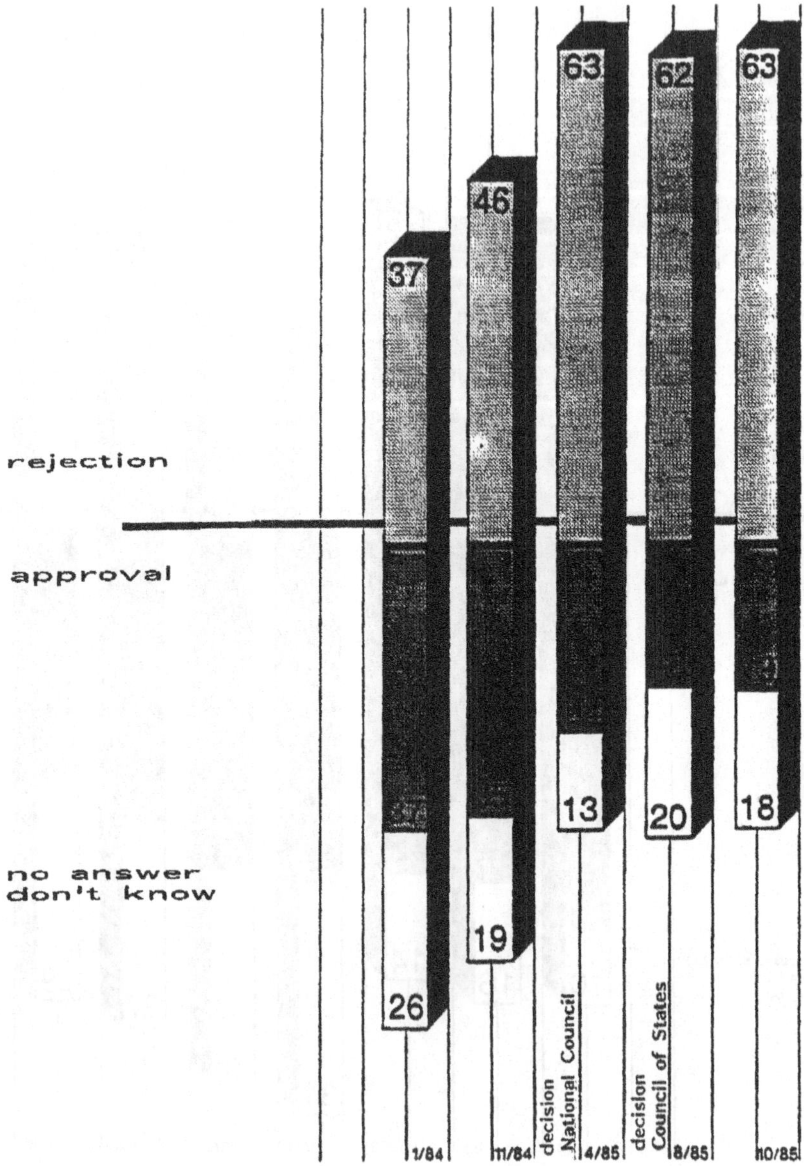

Fig. 2. Indirect question. How do you think the majority of the Swiss citizens will vote?

has to remember when campaigning: the first flow of information often has a negative impact. This is the statistical confirmation of what people feel when they are speaking of the sleeping dog which, in their eyes, one should let die. Personally, although I admit that, in the short range, once the dog is awake, it can of course be more aggressive and cause more trouble than

Fig. 3. Opinion poll November 1984.

Arguments against the abolishment of animal trials	
Endangers medical progress	55%
Endangers cancer research and research aimed at fighting other dangerous diseases	52%
Makes medicaments unsafe	48%
Means abolishment of all animal experimentation	43%
Endangers research in Switzerland	43%
Endangers our health care	40%

a sleeping one, I am against letting them die. If I wake them up, I am the first to have a chance to tell them what I know. If I let them sleep, the day they wake up by themselves, they may no longer listen to me!

Anyway, after a short period of worsening and a longer period of slow progress in our favour, we ended up with a positive result, very close to the result of the referendum.

The second question one has to check by doing opinion polls is the quality, pertinence and impact of the arguments. One of the keys of communication with the public is to concentrate on the best arguments and repeat them in many forms.

As Fig. 3 shows, the best argument for animal trials is the need for research aimed at fighting the most frightening diseases among us. This, in fact, has been our permanent argument, even if we did not forget two or three of the other ones.

The tools for such a campaign are many. First, you must publish a lot of material: booklets, short papers mailed to every body, advertising in the newspapers, posters, films and videos. We did all of this, under the umbrella of a committee called Committee for Research and Health. Moreover, and this has been of utmost importance, many of the health professionals produced their own material, such as a paper distributed by doctors and veterinarians to their patients (or 'patients' owners) as well as posters hung up by veterinarians on the walls and doors of their surgery.

In two towns, Geneva and Lausanne, professors, assistants and the staff working in biological research had the courage to go canvassing in the streets and speak directly to the people: a revolution in a very quiet country and for professions which are considered rather introverted. The weight the remarkable unanimity among all these professions carried with the citizens cannot be stressed enough.

Another problem, of course, was the press. In fact, it was not such a difficult one, because we had one enormous advantage: we had facts and figures to give them, while our opponents had nothing but vague or unfounded accusations which were not difficult to contest, so that we were credible and interesting for the press, while the antivivisectionists were not.

Pictures were a problem. At the beginning, we saw many old pictures in the press showing awful things, but never giving concrete information. We ourselves produced a large series of pictures, including not only harmless ones, but always with a precise telling what was being done to the animals, in which labs of which town, when and to which purpose. We sent them to the press and asked them not to publish these pictures without our legend. They did so and the other old and awful pictures simply disappeared.

We gave a lot of information to the press. In fact, within two years, there were about a dozen press conferences organized by several institutes, universities, hospitals and pharmaceutical companies, showing animal trials, their aim and their results. It had a major impact.

I say show and I would like to emphasize this word. Provided you carry out sound, correct and humane animal trials, which I consider obvious for any normal woman or man in research, you do not have to be afraid of having people from outside coming in and looking at what you do. During the last phase of the campaign, we invited as many clubs, associations, schools, etc. as possible to visit the laboratories in our industry, and it was always a relief for these visitors to see how we treat the animals. Many of the visitors, having previously been subject to the influence of antivivisectionists, were angry with our adversaries because they felt they had previously been lied to.

On the 2nd December 1985, the Swiss citizens voted and defeated the negative proposal by more than 70% against less than 30%. A big victory for biomedical research.

Unfortunately, we won a battle, not the war. The national Association for the Protection of Animals, which had been against abolishing animal trials, naturally had some problems with a part of its members. They decided to launch their own proposal, which does not go quite as far as prohibition, but would, if accepted, be dangerous for research, mainly fundamental research. It has more chance of being accepted, since it is less radical and is supported by a well-established, generally respected association, quite different from the fanatical groups which had launched the first one.

In other words, we are again engaged in a battle, ending in a referendum which will probably take place in 1991. But that's another story.

To come back to the first campaign, I should like to sum up our experience as follows:

- be happy if you presently have to work under severe legal conditions. It will help you to demonstrate that there is no need for abolition;
- produce as much information as you can on biomedical research, its successes in the past and the need for further progress against the severest illnesses, e.g. cancer, multiple sclerosis and AIDS;
- above all, open your doors, be visible, speak openly, show what you do!

In one sentence, my conclusion is that the only way for science to resist antivivisectionism (and to win other battles) is to be transparent. It is time-consuming, but it can be life-saving, not only for yourself, but also for millions of patients.

Experimentation and the law

JEAN-MARC VARAUT
Lawyer at the Court of Paris, Paris, France

All civilisations are concerned to protect animals, especially those living side by side with man. Some civilisations have gone beyond man's duty towards all living creatures and worship them as gods. But it is only lately that legislation has intervened to protect animals under the criminal law. In France, the first germ of a specific penal law appears to go back as far as 1791. Under that law people were held criminally liable for *maliciously* killing or wounding livestock or guard dogs. Then again, *maliciousness* was the essential factor constituting the crime of poisoning animals belonging to others provided by the 1910 Penal Code. The Grammont Law in 1850 was the first to introduce the idea of protecting animals against cruelty for their own sake. This law was extended in 1963. Since then improper treatment of animals has constituted a minor offence punishable by a fine or a short term of imprisonment (R 40), and poisoning or acts of cruelty are indictable offences (articles 452 to 454-1 of the Penal Code). Article 454 applies to people carrying out experiments or scientific or experimental research on animals without complying with the applicable regulations.

Under French positive law all animals are now protected against acts of cruelty. Although in fact the Penal Code only refers to domestic animals or animals kept in captivity, the Law of 10th July 1976 relating to the protection of nature and in consequence of fauna, deals with the keeping of protected non-domestic species of animals. But wild animals living freely in the wild are excluded from this protection, and this applies to game.

Accordingly, the aim of the criminal law is to punish *cruelty*, that is to say unnecessary or excessive suffering caused deliberately and gratuitously for the purpose of the satisfaction that some people obtain from suffering or death. Therefore, for such acts to be classified as crimes subject to trial before the criminal court, there has to be a perverted intention resembling sadism and acts exceeding the bounds of brutality – real acts of torture. Apart from these, such acts are classed as wrongful treatment, and thus are offences subject to trial by the police court. Examples are attaching a saucepan to a cat's tail, striking a cow that has fallen to force it to get up, or abandoning a dog on a roadside with its head and paws tied up.. It is thus evident that

S. Garattini (ed.), The Importance of Animal Experimentation for Safety and Biomedical Research, 35–38.

it is necessary for there to be a deliberate intention, and a finding of maliciousness; in addition, the offender has to have acted *needlessly*.

It is this idea of *need* which leads us on to experiments and scientific research carried out on live animals. A Decree dated 9th February 1968 lies behind articles R 24 - 14 to R 24–31 of the Penal Code which sanction failure to comply with the regulations relating to experiments or research on animals for the purpose of human or animal health or for teaching.

On 19th October 1987, ten ministers signed a new decree which added further rules to this strict but reasonable regulation, increasing the number of authorities, authorisations, notifications, justifications, prohibitions, inspections and training and whose aim or effect is to exclude animals from biological research laboratories in disregard of the radical progress achieved over the past fifty years. Yet pharmacological, toxicological and pharmacokinetic studies on animals have contributed to the progress which is evidenced by the fall in infant mortality and the considerable increase in life expectancy. Today Pasteur's experiments on rabies would have been deemed criminal offences subject to trial by the criminal court. And it is forgotten that the tragic thalidomide case, which is still cited, would never have happened if the drug had been administered to other species of animals than rats, which unfortunately were not affected by this product. Thalidomide is the best example of the absolute necessity for some experimentation on animals. I have submitted this decree to the *Conseil d'Etat* [the highest administrative court and advisory body to the government in matters of legislation], in that this excessive, finicky and absurd regulation interferes with the *freedom of scientific research* linked to human rights to health, scientific progress and teaching which make up the third generation of Human Rights. The notion of strict necessity which was the precondition for authorisation of experiments or scientific research has thus been called into question by a decree which increases the problems of authorising experiments, controlling the actual individual experimenters, and placing establishments, particularly pharmaceutical laboratories, under strict surveillance. One example of this is: people who have been criminally convicted or disciplined '*for acts contrary to honour or integrity*' (article 10, paragraph 3) cannot be experimenters. This devolution of jurisdiction to the Authorities is also an interference in the free exercise of professional activities. The 'Nanny' State wishes to play the rôle of Headmaster. Doctors have become disqualified adults under the guardianship of government officials.

This regulation is an expression in regulatory form of the present-day confusion in values. One can only approve the modern concern for ecology. The thin film of air, water and life on the surface of the earth has to be protected against the assaults threatening it. It is essential that mastery of the earth which has become the will for power does not destroy the earth. Serious and permanent disturbance of man's environment would call into question the future of mankind itself. In view of man's worldwide heritage, the 'good husbandman' has new obligations which should make him consider his heritage in time and space, its preservation and transmission from a different point of view. Man has added a technosphere to the biosphere, which is an extension of it and which, according to Julian Huxley can be expressed as '*the being's ability to dominate his environment and make himself independent of it*' but which must not destroy the environment in which the being develops. Although in Descartes' prophetic words science makes us '*masters and possessors of nature*', this is not so that *Homo sapiens*, or to use Descartes' term '*man capax scientiae*', since become '*Homo faber*', according to Bergson's famous expression, becomes criminal man. On the contrary the human race is the heir and bearer of the evolution of creation.

But creation has its order and its hierarchy. Baby seals are not analogous to human babies; wild geese are simply wild geese. Confusion becomes total when it is proclaimed that *animals have rights*. The ambiguous expression 'the natural law' has made such a declaration possible. But there is no law in nature. The law exists where freedom and history meet. It is one of the dimensions of human existence. It expresses a model for human relationships in the form of laws, case law precedents, and institutions. For the law is not simply a mechanism of restrictions. It is prompted with the aim of order and driven by the goal of justice. Law is specifically human. Like art, it is the privilege of an organisational thought process. In the space between *Sein* – the incomprehensible fact of being – and *Sollen* – the bounds of obligation – it is a real creator of social order and justice. It is the regulator of human societies, which contains a large proportion of expediency; in other words constant adaptation enlivened by the embodiment of ideas. This is an entirely practical task which constantly demands to go beyond the bounds of nature by instituting an order that does not *exist*. The intersubjectivity that is the philosophical expression of this permanent construction is not letting nature take its course but going further than nature does.

There is therefore no such thing as animal rights. Animals are not subject to the law. It is a question of putting man first. Experimentation and scientific research on animals respond to a moral duty which is also a legal obligation: protecting human life and improving human health. Man has duties towards animals; research and experiments must not be grounds for acts of cruelty or freedom to act sadistically. *Necessity* is the point where man's right to health and his duty to respect the biosphere, its legitimacy and its limit meet. Animals do not have rights, but man has responsibilities towards them, although his first duties are to man.

Because, whether one likes it or not, the law involves a certain notion of human destiny, and is one of the instruments of the achievement of that destiny, it ought to be of service to scientific research and assist it in harvesting its fruits, and improving them constantly, rather than paralysing that research. Creation was not given to man once and for all. Creation is ongoing. Man is co-creator. Claude Bernard, who perhaps was not aware how close he was to Christian creation theology, said that by experimental medicine man became '*an actual artisan of creation*'. Although limits have to be placed on his desire for power, although these limits have to be fixed by a Penal Code, there can be no limits the power man can acquire over nature.

The upsurge in legislation which threatens to lead to the collapse of Europe's system of general law, based on a number of articles of the Treaty of Rome and the European Declaration of Human Rights and Fundamental Freedoms, is shown in these manifold Directives from a Europe of bureaucrats, which is not yet subject to any political power. This overabundance of sources of law, which is not giving any signs of drying up, is leading to the *devaluation* and *depreciation* of the law, to contempt of it, and its decline. Whereas everyone should be able to do what he has to do and what he wants, with what he is and what he has, on his own responsibility and subject to the sanctions of the criminal law, the increasing proliferation of legislation in all realms of society is leading to irresponsibility on the part of mankind and to invention lying fallow. Battle has commenced between the European Declaration of Human Rights and Domination by Symbol, Europe of the Judges and Europe of the Eurocrats. The European Council Directive of 24th November 1986 relating to the harmonization of Member states' legislative and administrative provisions and regulations with regard to the protection of animals used for experimental or other scientific purposes, is one of the symbols that shows that the regulatory protectorate of European officialdom is gaining ground. We shall be appealing to the *Europe of the Judges*.

Experimentation on animals: Animals as machines and animals as fetishes

JANINE CHANTEUR
University of Sorbonne, Paris, France

Experimentation on animals arouses intense emotions. Some refuse to discuss the grounds for such a practice: they believe that when it comes to protecting human health, no questions are to be asked which might delay research. Others, on the contrary, and among them the ecologists, maintain that the practice is totally unfounded in the scientific order and see in it one of the signs of the moral deterioration of western civilization. In fact, this is a concept which decides on its lack of utility or its utility without relying on any serious study.

A philosopher must think calmly, remembering that he is not a scientist, but he must also refrain from making any value judgements on the basis of inadequate reasoning. His task is to attempt to single out the principles which enable all parties to de-dramatize the debate and adopt a line of conduct which the law can enforce.

How does the philosopher confront the issue of experimentation on animals? And is his involvement legitimate?

The issue in the experimentation on animals is a voluntary action on the part of man on a living being of another species, decided upon to the benefit of his own species. In other words, in order to progress, the specifically human scientific and technical approach, in the case which interests us, is to have to utilize animals, as one would use things, to increase knowledge of disease, to find the means of preventing and curing it.

It is clear that applying this approach, man attributes himself a worth which is in no way comparable to that he grants animals. In order to protect himself, all means are good. That which is accepted in the realm of food and clothing, since meat and leather shoes have not yet been questioned, apparently becomes more serious in the realm of health, on account of the animals suffering, inevitable in certain experiments. Whence the problem the philosopher must inevitably tackle: does man have the right to experiment on animals, particularly when he cannot altogether eliminate their suffering? Does the maintenance of his life – at this cost – not eliminate the moral, even metaphysical meaning, that human life may have?

Before tackling possible answers, we must point out two things:

The first is that a form of veterinary medicine exists which relies on

S. Garattini (ed.), The Importance of Animal Experimentation for Safety and Biomedical Research, 39–46

medication which has necessarily been tested, either on other animals or, when care was first administered, on the diseased animal. But one must also ask the following question: are there priviledged animals (those that are loved by man or which bring in income – dogs, cats, sheep, cattle, etc.) and the mass of other animals, left to experimentation?

The second remark pertains to the Charter of Animal Rights. We all concur that it was not created by animals – and for good reason. And yet it cannot be compared to a charter of children's rights or a charter of rights for the handicapped, for they are fully-fledged human beings. That one is speaking on their behalf ensues from the logic of the definition of a human species which grants itself certain rights; the Charter of Animals Rights is therefore a projection, a transfer of that which is thought to suit the human, species to other species. But this is in fact a fallacy, because the declarations of human rights have (or at least should have) meaning only if those very men entitled to those rights acknowledge the inevitable corollary of rights – duties. The notion of rights, detached from the notion of duty, is devoid of meaning.

But animals never have duties. They can be trained to do or not to do something. Their behavior is never combined with reflection. A child's education includes a training aspect, but it warrants the term education only if the training aspect is entirely transcended in a continuous process of questioning and reviewing of each 'conditioning' imparted. Then only can one speak of a moral obligation and rights attached to it. No act of this type characterizes animals.

Let us return to the question we asked above, which the foregoing comments help us situate: does man, we wonder, have the right to experiment on animals, particularly when he cannot avoid making them suffer? We added: does the preservation of human life at this cost destroy the specifically human meaning of that life?

In an initial stage, we shall base the justification for experimentation, and therefore the right to experiment, on the irreducible difference between animal and man. In a second stage, we shall ask ourselves whether this difference does not in actual fact imply the duty to cease experimentations by virtue of considerations of a higher order. We shall then be at a stage where we must again justify the principle of the right to experiment and its limits. Lastly, we shall seek to determine the ideologies which more or less consciously underlie the form of protest developing at present.

In order to decide whether man can justifiably experiment on animals, at the risk of the latter's suffering, we must first of all single out the aim of experimentation. Here one purpose is to use animals, when other working methods are inadequate, in order to better clarify the evolution of a disease. When a member of the human species is ill, it is his body, in the first analysis, which is threatened. In a human being, disease undermines the animal – as testified to by many familiar expressions: 'the beast is ill...', and other sayings. To re-establish the health of the human animal, research calls upon other animals to be sacrificed, by making them suffer or even putting them to death.

This may seem paradoxical, even absurd or criminal. If we were speaking merely of the intervention of one animal or another animal, this would constitute no problem of rights, regardless of the nature of the intervention. Nor would it constitute a moral issue: the fact that a wolf makes a lamb suffer while eating it or that a dog breaks the hind quarters of a cat for no reason, and the cat takes hours dying in a state of atrocious suffering, is neither good nor bad.

On the other hand, the fact that a man inflicts suffering upon an animal with the intention of curing men or of assuaging their suffering constitutes a problem, because man is not merely an animal. Unlike the animal, man is a being for whom an action is never neutral. It is either good or bad, it has a value. Man is an animal who evaluates, who lends a meaning to his existence. This is why he poses the problem of the meaning and worth of experimentation on animals, while at the same time understanding that the very fact that he is asking himself this question distinguished him for ever from the animal and consequently implies his agreement that the treatment man reserves for man need not be the same he reserves for animals.

To save a man is a duty, because each man, despite his obvious moral shortcomings, is a center of ethical activity and because the condition which makes an ethical existence possible is the life of the body and, to the greatest extent possible, its wholeness and health.

This is why only man is capable of caring for the ill: he cares for man and sometimes also for animals. Animals are totally indifferent to suffering which is not theirs. The rescuing of others, such as by Saint-Bernards or other dogs in relation to their masters, is the result of training or habit, not a voluntary decision comparable to a duty. When one observes the suffering of a human mother at the bedside of a child with a terminal illness and that of an animal mother in the same situation, there is no possible comparison. The human mother can go so far as to offer her life for her child by asking, if necessary, to be the donor of a vital organ. An animal mother is not preoccupied with her offspring and may even spurn it.

This means that man has the duty to provide care, to man first of all above any other being. This is testified to by man's laws which punish the failure to assist persons in danger. Illness is a danger which can be fatal. Distress for the ill means urgency for the physician and requires that he has at his disposal the means of assuaging pain and of curing illness, to as great an extent as possible, at any cost except that of another human life. (With the exception of a case as above of a mother choosing to let her child live rather than herself or that of a human being risking and even losing his life to save the life of another. In both these cases, it is a question of evaluating, and value is still given to human life).

We can thus henceforth conclude that when the task is to save man (and therefore to enhance our knowledge of human biology, the etiology of disease, the most suitable medication), man has indefinite, in other words infinite, right on all that is not human, because it is his duty to care for man. All that is not human includes of course all animal species.

Does this mean that animals are to be linkened to a thing, more precisely to a machine, in accordance with Descartes' expression, in the 5th part of the Discours de la Méthode, which he reiterated in other works? Descartes, we recall, who separated thinking and expanse, the soul and the body, and denied animals both soul and thinking, defined animals as machines, robots, purely subject to the determinism of natural laws. However, if animal behavior escapes determinism only slightly, it is nonetheless true that animals are capable of suffering. The animal does not represent his suffering as man does, but it is unquestionably felt in a manner other than were it to be a mere mechanical effect. A machine has no feelings. Animals do. To liken animals to machines is one of the erroneous consequences of Cartesian dualism and strict rationalism which claims to give an account of life. An animal is not a robot, although he is determined. The mystery of life is not solved by natural science.

Does man have the right to inflict suffering, which is sometimes very great and useless, when the experiment has proved sterile, in order to seek the means of his own health? If animals are not things, does man have the right to treat them like things? And furthermore, should the question not be put the other way round: in face of a being weaker than oneself, who is incapable of putting up an effective resistance, is not man's duty exactly the opposite, i.e. to refrain from harming him? Experimentation would degrade what man holds as his essential difference: his capacity to distinguish good from bad, to act in a moral manner. It appears difficult to claim that animals – at least some of them – are man's friends while willingly subjecting them to suffering and death.

Have we perhaps reached a contradiction beyond which we cannot go? On the one hand, it is man's duty to care for man by all and any means, because human life is a value; on the other hand, an animal is a defenseless being capable of suffering, but he cannot be utilized like a thing for he is not inanimate?

As we can see, experimentation on animals is not an absolutely well-founded right, regardless of the modalities. Because man is an ethical being and because this is his irreplaceable value, he can neither forego caring for man, for this is his most pressing duty, nor can he refuse to consider animal suffering, for this too is his duty. The apparent aporia calls for us to go beyond it because the conflict of two duties is not to be defined according to equal forces. In all circumstances, a man is worth more than an animal, but the animal exists and suffers. This contradiction can only be resolved by a clear condition to experimentation: animal suffering is bearable only when it remains the sole and truly the sole means of scientific research, with a view to ensuring human health.

In other words, the ethical order is not self-sufficient; it requires legal constraint, but the law has no meaning unless it foregoes pressure and passion, and ensures first of all the protection of human beings. Protection of health and a more subtle protection against improper conduct by anyone who invokes health as a pretext and believes he is entitled to do anything. Only in this way are animals protected but, one must agree, as a second intent, as the first is reserved to man who, as a victim of bewildering masochism, might otherwise promulgate laws contrary to the well-being of all.

We are only too aware moreover of the degree to which men are devious when it comes to transgressing the law; experimentation would 'fly the Panama flag', if you pardon the expression. This means that without the least legal guarantee, laboratories would hasten to expatriate their research workes to work under skies less particular when it comes to laws. The epitome would be that research can be expected in coming years to produce a cure of vaccination against one of the incurable diseases plaguing the world. Thus the transgressor of the laws of his own country would be humanity's savior and receive the Nobel Prize! Who wants to play angel...

It is nonetheless legitimate to be more exacting and to push our questioning further. Have we not calmed our consciences a little too hastily, by giving human life a price which it would certainly have as the means of its own meaning, but which owes to modern thinking the idea that the human being exceeds all other beings, therefore animals, because he is a center of evaluation and significance. Assuredly, an animal is part of an order of things which he does not question, which he does not transform, because he does not think about it. He is content to live in the present, while man stands at a distance in relation to his world, he thinks about it and upon it. There is certainly no comparison between the dearth of animal representations and the incredible wealth of human representations. It is perhaps even less arrogant than it appears to claim than man is the 'master and possessor of nature', as Descartes felt confident in doing.

But if, on the contrary, man too is inscribed in the world's order, not just as the things and animals which are subject to the laws of nature, but in a cosmic order in which it would be his duty to seek the meaning, which would not depend on him, to know the meaning without curtailing it, while assuming the minerals, plants, beasts and other man, in an ascent toward the principle which, in its transparency, renders inteligible the multiplicity of the world. Is such a metaphysical vision of the world's redemption by an at last clairvoyant mankind compatible with the suffering inflicted upon animals, in order to cure the life of the human body? This is what some opponents of scientific research – among the purest and generally the least violent – ask themselves and certain techniques hardly inclined to question their practices. The poet and philosopher, Angelus Silesius, perpetuating a long tradition, spoke in these words to he whose mission was unification and love:

> 'Man, all feel love for you,
> There is great haste around you
> All rush toward you to reach God...
> If you possess the Creator, then all run after you,
> Man, angel, sun and moon, air, fire, earth and brook'.

Animals, needless to say, along with plants, are included in the evocation of the earth.

As for myself, I am tempted to hark to this voice which casts an entirely fresh light on human achievement. How, while remaining coherent, shall I henceforth tackle the concrete problem that preoccupies us? Well, I shall take the risk of not changing the conclusions we had reached, but I must provide some justification for them.

If it is true that man is the essential mediation between what one might call the sky and the earth, and if he is called upon to work toward a metaphysical reconciliation of all creation, the life of his body is no longer an end in itself, but the duty to preserve it always constitutes the necessary condition of a cosmic end.

What then becomes of the almost Francescan fraternity with animals, one wonders, if he does not hesitate to sacrifice them for his profit? It appears to me what we must more than ever be wary of the temptation – all the more dangerous as it has taken on the aspect of a necessary consequence implicit in the metaphysical mission of the human species – to save the world by gathering its scattered elements, instead of by using them selfishly. The temptation is to believe that we have reached the end of history, to imagine man's access to a reinstated nature, as though he had already reached the light. Again, however, we come up against the contradiction: must we, on the one hand, abandon the hosts of men suffering the misery of their tortured bodies, in the name of a coming fraternity of all creation? Or must we care for man and sacrifice animals, as though we were abandoning the memory of our ties with them?

Decidedly, all the channels of reflection lead man to go beyond: finite create, he is lost if he thinks he can act in this world without coming up against the duty which is as necessary as it is often painful to choose man, as long as the history of mankind lasts; but also, if he forgets that the accomplishment of a duty does not confer all rights upon man. As soon as the means of experimentation accompanied by suffering for the animal can be abandoned without harm to man, it must be abandoned, even if it means working harder. On the other hand, as long as it is the sole recourse against human suffering, man must have the courage to use it, while attempting to hasten the time when it will become useless, because man and animals are not meant, in a cosmic vision, to be used by each other, as one uses an inanimate object. It is an extravagant dream to imagine that man, in the living conditions which exist on this hearth, can avoid being obliged to choose. We cannot have everything, the satisfaction of accomplishing our duty toward man while also keeping our hands clean when it comes to animals.

Once again, we find ourselves up against the limits of what the law must make clear, but we have met one more requirement: by using animals to assuage man's pain, research workers must remember that their work is good when it helps cure, and better still when, with an eye on the cosmic meaning of the human adventure, they strive never to employ an animal when other means are available. Thus is observed the hierarchy into which beast and man, different by nature and vocation, fit. Thus the ever latent temptation to abandon men by lending man a stature which is not historically his is avoided.

In fact, when one looks at things realistically, it is not difficult to discover the goals set by protest. Behind the groups, which cater more to a wounded sentimentality than to a true metaphysical aspiration, what do we find? For most, though not for all, first of all there is the desire to protect themselves from the hard confrontation with human illness, suffering and death, and at the same time the desire to flee the uncertain relation men have with others. The animal becomes a 'fetish', easy to defend, because he never questions the significance attributed to him. Man is more difficult to approach and the feelings he provokes are more distressing. Men, one must agree, easily discourage the interest it is our duty to show for them for reasons we have tried to set out. They are not good and fear, their most familiar companion, inspires in them aggressive conduct or vainglory which are not good incentives to decoding the meaning they nonetheless bear. Animals do not hide any enigmas and their protection, for those who do not have the courage to defend men, is often an easy alibi.

Another, more dangerous reason inspires certain protesters against experimentation, and among the most violent. Nature, it is obvious, is not egalitarian. It made men themselves so different from one another that it is an aberration to attempt to see the same aptitudes in every man - which in no way means that they do not have the same human dignity. Egalitarian ideology is inseparable from a levelling off which necessarily works from the bottom for the misfortune of all, above all the most deprived. By denying man, in the name of animal suffering, improperly likened to human suffering, the right to experiment on animals within the strict limits of the prevention and curing of disease, do we not insidiously identify man with that in him which is least human: nature, subject to the mechanism of determinism? We readily admit that the latter is more complex in man that in animals, but the difference becomes a difference of degree not of nature. One easily recognizes the ideology working behind the manipulation of distressed groups in whom it is sufficient to flatter the 'kind' feelings in order to lead them on. Placing man and animal on the same level makes it easier for us to erase the differences which resisted among men, to disorient beings who are less and less certain of their definition and of their vocation as men.

This is also an excellent method for slowing down research in 'liberal' countries, even if we do worse than they do in secret. One can see that behind a problem that has been termed '*humanitarian*', there are indeed a number of questions which involve human beings. It would not be courageous to evade the answers, either by sinking into in a dogmatic approach, or by declaring that they cannot be found. They certainly warrant a subtle presentation. But it is the sign of both the finite condition and the greatness of man to take his defense while assuming his full responsibilities when he makes animals one of his ultimate instruments, within the limits of law, of his struggle against scourges which have no respect for human suffering.

The law, however well devised, does not guide the research worker's hand in his work. It determines a framework inside which each of us, in line with the ethical and metaphysical interest he feels in life, remains free to decide the decency of his gestures. In all human things evil, as Socrates said, 'runs after us faster than death'. The danger of cruelty on the one hand and on the other hand that of succumbing to superfluous scruples lie in wait for the research worker. Human life is like walking on a razor's edge. Assisted or contained by legality, confronted with a problem such as experimentation on animals, it cannot receive its meaning from the outside. It is up to man and man alone, at grips with habit, prejudice, daring, but also with the mournful assaults of a bad conscience which never stops heaping ashes on his head, to determine his actions, in his own undoubtedly legitimate favor.

RECENT PROGRESS OF MEDICINE REQUIRING THE USE OF ANIMALS

The role of animal experiments in pharmacological brain research

ARVID CARLSSON
Department of Pharmacology, University of Gothenburg, Gothenburg, Sweden

Introduction

Technical advances in recent years have opened up a variety of possibilities for investigating physiological and biochemical mechanisms on isolated *in vitro* systems of cultured cells or cell components, such as enzymes, receptors, second messenger systems and carrier molecules involved in transport across cell membranes. Such studies are carried out at an increasing level of sophistication, utilizing the most recent advances in biotechnology. Some of these procedures compete favorably with traditional *in vivo* techniques, using animals, in terms of cost as well as time. Needless to say, they are especially welcome from the ethical point of view, since they reduce the number of experiments that have to be performed on the whole animal.

As a consequence of this highly satisfactory development there is a growing belief, especially among laymen, that experiments on whole animals can soon be done away with altogether. It has been argued that the continued use of animal experiments is entirely due to the slowness of the scientific community in assimilating recent technical advances. This is a serious misunderstanding. If we wish to make progress in our understanding of body functions and utilize this knowledge in the diagnosis, treatment and prevention of diseases in humans and animals, animal experiments will still be essential. If regulatory procedures are implemented that will make animal experimentation increasingly difficult, the dramatic progress in current biomedical research and its clinical application will soon be brought to a standstill. Millions of human beings will thus be deprived of therapeutic and prophylactic procedures serving to reduce suffering of various kinds. To enforce such restrictions would be foolish and unethical.

The field of CNS pharmacology can offer numerous examples of the decisive role of animal experimentation. Below a few of these, taken from the author's personal experience, will be discussed.

S. Garattini (ed.), The Importance of Animal Experimentation for Safety and Biomedical Research, 49–56.

The discovery of antipsychotic agents and their mode of action

In terms of suffering schizophrenia ranks high among human disorders. The discovery of the modern antipsychotic agents in the 1950s has not eliminated this scourge but has dramatically improved the possibilities for millions of schizophrenics, who would otherwise be condemned to asylums, to lead a reasonably normal life. Chlorpromazine first attracted attention among a series of antihistaminic agents, intended for use in allergic disorders, by its unusual sedative action on animals. This property finally led to trials in psychotic patients and to the discovery of its remarkable effect on the complex symptomatology of schizophrenia [1]. There was not nothing in the pharmacological profile of this agent apart from its unusual calming effect on animals that would have suggested a trial in psychiatric patients.

Needless to say, the mode of action of a compound with such remarkable effects on the human mind is an issue of considerable interest. This problem could only be solved by analyzing the biochemical changes occurring in the brains of animals treated with the drug. These changes led to the concept of dopamine as a key neurotransmitter involved in the action of antipsychotic agents. Only later could in vitro experiments be done to demonstrate the molecular effect [2].

But could this problem not have been tackled using cell cultures? The answer is definitely no. We have to remember that the number of dopaminergic nerve cells in the human brain is about one million, as compared to a total number of brain neurons of about 10 to 100 billions. The proportions are roughly the same in other mammalian brains. A cell culture of brain neurons would not be likely to contain any dopaminergic neurons or synapses, and thus this specific action of chlorpromazine would be missed altogether.

Breakthrough in the understanding and treatment of a major neurological disorder

The study of the actions of antipsychotic agents in animals led to another important discovery. In 1957 Courvoisier [3] described a strange action of these agents on animal behavior. When treated with large doses of these drugs the animals became immobile and could be placed and remained in the most awkward positions. Later it was realized that this condition had a counterpart in man: so-called extrapyramidal side effects, among them Parkinsonism. When Courvoisier described these effects in 1957 nobody had the slightest idea about the mechanism involved. But about one month later the experiment leading to an understanding of this mechanism was performed. It was found that this condition of extreme immobility, which is called catalepsy, could be dramatically antagonized by the injection of DOPA. This in turn led to the identification of dopamine as an agonist in its own right in the brain and to the proposal that Parkinsonism and Parkinson's disease are brought about by an insufficient function of dopamine. As a consequence, Austrian workers examined the brains of diseased Parkinson patients and found reduced levels of dopamine. Finally this led to the introduction of L-DOPA in the treatment of Parkinson's disease (see ref. [2]). The severe suffering of millions of human beings could thus be alleviated. We have here an example where the observation of drug effects on animal behavior led to a break-through in the understanding and treatment of a debilitating disorder. There seemed to be no alternative way of making this discovery. Based on these discoveries research is now aiming at clarifying the etiology of Parkinson's disease and designing strategies for its prevention.

The discovery of receptor subtypes: New avenues of selectivity in elucidating brain functions and in development of novel therapeutic principles

In the course of biological evolution and natural selection nature turns out to possess incredible ingenuity. Thus a given neurotransmitter will usually be utilized for an astonishing variety of purposes. To achieve this the evolution of different receptor molecules recognizing one and the same endogenous agonist often prove appropriate. The medicinal chemist can exploit the existence of receptor subtypes to design molecules with affinity for only one of the subtypes. He will thus surpass nature in terms of selective manipulation. In fact, the discovery of receptor subtypes is often based on the advent of such chemical tools.

In vitro methods based on binding of ligands to receptor molecules or on the coupling of receptors to enzymes or ion channels have proved extremely valuable in basic receptor research and have to some extent replaced classical approaches measuring the performance of isolated tissues or whole animals. However, *in vitro* systems will never be able to replace animal experiments entirely.

The following example may serve to illustrate the role of animal experiments in receptor research. When one of the serotonin receptor subtypes, called 5-HT-1A receptors [4], is stimulated by a selective agonist, certain behavioral changes, which are believed to predict anxiolytic activity in humans, are observed in animals. At the same time there is a decrease in blood pressure. For the purpose of drug development the separation of the two effects would seem desirable. To achieve this the medicinal chemist prepares series of new molecules which differ from the previously known 5-HT-1A agonists in various substituents or ring structures. The aim is to find compounds which act on behavior, but not on blood pressure, and *vice versa*. If the approach proves successful, *in vitro* experiments can be started, aiming to isolate the sub-subtypes of 5-HT-1A receptors, engaged in the behavioral and hypotensive action, respectively. Many efforts of this type are now being made in academic circles and drug industry research. Only the future will tell which are going to be successful. There is no doubt, however, that this type of endeavor is promising and will result in the development of valuable new therapeutic agents.

Unravelling the physiological basis of the mind

Modern imaging techniques have opened up astounding possibilities for investigating the brain, not only morphologically but also regarding its biochemistry and physiology. For example, the oxygen consumption and metabolic activity of various brain regions can be measured in human beings, using non-invasive techniques. The ability of specific neurons to form and accumulate their neurotransmitters can be studied. Likewise, the distribution of the receptors which mediate the message from one neuron to another can be visualized and quantified [5]. Using such techniques, it is now possible to observe how the brain responds to various stimuli or when it is challenged to increase mental activity [6].

To develop these imaging techniques animal experiments are necessary. For example, radioactive precursors or ligands for receptor studies have to be tried out in animals before they can be used in man. On the whole, such studies in humans benefit enormously from preparatory work on animals.

The human mind is of course extremely complex, but through these various techniques it is no longer beyond reach for investigation. Even here molecular studies using various *in vitro* techniques are indispensable. However, the final analysis will have to be carried out on the intact brain. It appears that mental activity is not strictly localized in a limited area, such as the cerebral cortex, but requires a complex interaction between the cortex and several subcortical structures, for example the striatum, the thalamus, the hypothalamus, and the lower brain stem with its important reticular formation [7]. It goes without saying that this interaction must be investigated in the intact brain.

The vertebrate brain has undergone a fascinating evolution from the most primitive fish stage all the way up to man. To investigate the brain at different levels of sophistication gives many useful insights. The brains of mammals are basically similar to the human brain, though generally much simpler. The study of the brains of lower mammals yields an enormous amount of information, useful for the final analysis of human brain function.

Knowledge about the human mind has considerable value in itself. The human brain is perhaps the most sophisticated product of millions of years of biological evaluation but is nevertheless far from perfect. To better understand its limitations and possibilities is an urgent need. Most of the serious problems in this world are man-made and can thus be regarded as an expression of the lack of perfection of the human brain. By learning more about brain function we can design new strategies to improve human behavior.

Mental disorders play a dominating role in human pathology. The new insights into brain function that are now emerging will no doubt lead to new strategies for prevention and treatment of major mental disorders, such as schizophrenia, affective disorders and dementia. Within the next one or two decades we can expect remarkable developments in this area.

The aging brain: A rapidly growing problem in our society

No cell in the body can escape the aging process. The nerve cells of the brain are especially vulnerable and if they are lost, they cannot be replaced. The number of aging people is rapidly growing. To find measures to alleviate the functional losses and suffering caused by aging is one of the most urgent tasks of biomedical research today. Considerable progress is now being made in the understanding of mechanisms underlying neuronal degeneration.

One such mechanism is based on the fact that excessive release of excitatory transmitters, for example glutamate, may induce a dangerously high level of stimulation, resulting in cell damage and death [8]. Such release may be induced by insufficient reuptake of released transmitter following ischemia. Agents are now being developed which block the receptors involved, the so-called NMDA receptors, and which have thus been found to protect animals from neuronal death induced by ischemia. One such agent, namely Mk-801, is now undergoing clinical trials. Mk-801 may not prove to be the final answer, on account of possible mental side effects, but the approach is clearly promising [9].

Another factor involved in neuronal degeneration may be excessive intracellular concentrations of calcium ions. Such accumulation may, in fact, be induced by excitatory amino acids; the two mechanisms mentioned so far may thus be interrelated. So-called calcium channel blockers have accordingly been able to afford some protection against ischemic neuronal damage.

A third factor of interest in this context is free oxygen radicals. These highly cytotoxic entities may be formed in excessive amounts if the protective system of antioxidants should fail. Again, ischemic conditions and hypoglycemia may lead to depletion of antioxidants and thus to accumulation of cytotoxic oxygen radicals. Animal experiments are needed to further clarify the role of this mechanism as well as the ones mentioned previously in disorders caused by premature neuronal degeneration.

Toxic factors in our environment may induce neuronal degeneration. An interesting model substance in this context is MPTP (1-methyl-4-phenyl-1,2,3,6-tetrahydropyridine, see ref. [10]). This agent is unintentionally formed in an illicit synthetic process to prepare a heroin-like compound. When given to primates, including man, and to mice, but not to rats, it causes a highly selective neuronal degeneration, involving almost exclusively dopaminergic neurons. As a consequence, the typical picture of Parkinson's disease is induced. In humans the condition is essentially irreversible. Several tragic cases of Parkinsonism induced by this agent have been observed among drug addicts in the U.S. MPTP is an instructive example of the difficulties involved in establishing the safety of candidate drugs. Obviously cell cultures would not reveal this highly selective neuronal toxicity. Intact animals will have to be used. To discover neuronal damage, the animals must survive several days. Rats, which are often used in drug safety testing, are not susceptible to this neurotoxic agent. The existence of this type of neurotoxic mechanism shows that animal experiments will probably always have to be performed in drug safety investigations. Besides, MPTP is an interesting model substance in the search for toxic agents in our environment.

Other research activities of considerable interest in the study of neurodegenerative conditions deal with nerve growth factors, which are now being discovered in considerable numbers [16]. Lack of such factors may be the causes of some neurodegenerative conditions. In fact, certain animal experiments suggest that the administration of gangliosides may provide some protection against neurodegenerative factors, and such compounds are currently undergoing trials in humans.

Growth factors may possible be needed to ensure successful nerve cell grafts, for instance in Parkinson's disease. Transplantations have been tried in a limited number of cases of this disorder, though not yet with undoubtedly positive results. However, in animal models of Parkinson's disease grafting has turned out to be remarkably successful. Obviously further animal experiments are needed to clarify why grafting in human disease has not yet been equally successful.

In summary, research aiming to develop new treatment and prevention strategies in neurodegenerative disorders is in a very active and promising phase. Further progress in this area will be highly dependent on animal experimentation.

The suffering induced by animal experiments, viewed in a broader perspective

The information of the public concerning animal experiments is often extremely lopsided. It is generally supplied by animal movement organisations, whose propaganda has proved remarkably successful.

In most of the experiments of the type described the degree of suffering of experimental animals has been slight or moderate. Many experiments simply involve the injection of pharmacological agents with specific sites of action in the brain and observations of the behavioral changes induced. In cases where surgical procedures are performed, the animals are almost invariably anesthetized. Only in rare cases is only local anesthesia adequate.

When evaluating the ethical problems involved in scientific animal experiments, it is useful to compare suffering caused by the handling of animals in our society in general. In this context we have to bear in mind that the need for animals for non-scientific purposes is very limited in a modern society. Animal food products are not needed. In fact the general health of the population would probably improve, if anything, if we abstained entirely from the consumption of animal food products. Neither do we need animal products for our clothing. Obviously, sport fishing, hunting and horse-racing can easily be disposed of. In summary, practically all animal handling, apart from scientific animal experiments, is simply carried out for our pleasure and convenience. Nevertheless, this handling involves a great variety of animal suffering. In the case of animal experiments, the ethical rule is that the degree of animal suffering should be weighed against the importance of the experiment from the scientific point of view, keeping in mind that the ultimate goal of the research is to alleviate and prevent human suffering. In a committee of animal ethics an experiment involving animal suffering, even of moderate degree, would probably not be approved if the experiment was not judged to serve this purpose. Paradoxically, animal handling leading even to rather severe suffering is allowed in our society, provided the purpose is not scientific. For example, if an experiment were proposed, where the animals were whipped frenetically in order to induce a maximum of motor activity, the experiment would probably be turned down. But this is an every-day experience in horse racing. Or if an experiment were proposed where foreign objects were introduced at random into the bodies of unanesthetized animals, and where the animals were left to survive regardless of the suffering induced, this would certainly not be approved. But again this is an every-day event in hunting.

Concluding remarks

The discovery of the antipsychotic antidepressant drugs in the 1950s has had a great impact on brain research. Animal experiments on the mode of action of these agents played a decisive role for the establishment of chemical neurotransmission as the fundamental principle for communication between brain cells. This in turn has revolutionized brain research, which is now largely guided by this principle. As a result, the suffering of millions of human beings with Parkinson's disease and other neuropsychiatric disorders has been alleviated.

Continued work in this field will in all likelihood lead to an increased understanding of brain function and to new principles for therapy and, in certain cases, prophylaxis in major CNS disorders such as schizophrenia, affective disorders and neurogeriatric conditions, e.g. dementia and Parkinson's disease.

Basic brain research aims in part to clarify physiological and pathogenetic mechanisms at the molecular level. This work can often be done using *in vitro* systems obtained from brain tissue of animals and deceased human beings. However, the final analysis, serving to establish the relevance of molecular mechanisms for brain function, wll have to be done on animals as well as on humans.

Another important aspect of brain research aims at clarifying the brain's function as a system in which different regions, such as the cerebral cortex, the basal ganglia, the thalamus, hypothalamus and the lower brain stem interact in a complex manner. This type of analysis, which is absolutely essential for the understanding of brain function and brain disorders, will have to be done on intact animals and humans.

For similar reasons intact animals will always have to be employed in work aiming to establish the safety of potential therapeutic agents.

When dealing with ethical aspects of animal experimentation, we must aim at uniform principles encompassing all animal handling in our society.

References

1. Deniker P (1983) Discovery of the clinical use of neuroleptics. In: Parnham, MJ, Bruinvels, J (Eds) *Discoveries in Pharmacology*. Vol. 1: Psycho- and Neuro-Pharmacology, Elsevier, Amsterdam/New York/Oxford, pp 163–180
2. Carlsson A (1987) Perspectives on the discovery of central monoaminergic neurotransmission. *Ann Rev Neurosci* 10: 19–40
3. Courvoisier S, Ducrot R, Julou L (1957) Nouveaux aspects expérimentaux de l'activité centrale des dérives de la phénothiazine. In: Garattini, S, Ghetti, V (Eds) *Psychotropic Drugs*, Elsevier, Amsterdam/New York, pp 373–391
4. Dourish CT, Ahlenius S, Hutson PH (1987) *Brain 5-HT-1A Receptors*, Ellis Horwood, Chichester, England, pp 1–306
5. Farde L (1987) Dopamine Receptor Characteristics in the Living Human Brain, Thesis, Karolinska Institute, Stockholm, Sweden, pp 1–40
6. Roland PE (1987) Changes in brain blood flow and oxidative metabolism during mental activity. *News in Physiol Sci* 2: 120–124
7. Carlsson A (1988) The current status of the dopamine hypothesis of schizophrenia. *Neuropsychopharmacology* 1: 179–203
8. Cotman CW, Monaghan DT, Ganong AH (1988) Excitatory amino acid neurotransmission: NMDA receptors and Hebb-type synaptic plasticity. *Ann Rev Neurosci* 11: 61–80
9. Iversen LL (1988) Test models and new directions in dementia research. In: Casey, DE, Christensen, AV (Eds) *Psychopharmacology: Current Trends*. Springer, Berlin/Heidelberg, pp 196–203
10. Kopin IJ (1987) Neurotoxins affecting biogenic aminergic neurons. In: Meltzer, HY (Ed) *Psychopharmacology. The Third Generation of Progress*. Raven Press, New York, pp 351–358

Regeneration of the nervous system

ALFREDO GORIO[1,2] and FLAMINIO CATTABENI[1]
[1] *Institute of Pharmacological Sciences, and*
[2] *Istituto Scientifico H. San Raffaele, Milan, Italy*

Introduction

Medical and scientific interest in the processes of degeneration and regeneration of the nervous system has been increasing gradually but significantly in recent years. This stems from social, medical and scientific grounds. The frequency of degenerative disorders of the nervous system, including acute traumatic and ischemic insults, is steadily rising and the now routine application of molecular biology techniques to such problems opens new avenues of investigation raising hopes for new effective drug development and therapeutic strategies.

The international demographic pattern shows unequivocably how the population of elderly has grown: in the United States the number of people 65 years of age or over rose from 3.1 million in 1900 to 26 million in 1980. The percentage of the elderly population, therefore, jumped from 4.1 to 11.3 and in the year 1990 it is expected to reach about 13%. Current estimates indicate that in the future the developed countries will be populated by an even higher percentage of elderly, about 30% of the population reaching 80 years of age.

The occurrence of degenerative neurological disorders such as Alzheimer's disease is directly correlated with advanced age, so that the risk of having such a disease would reach 20% among the elderly. No other risk factors have been associated with Alzheimer's disease. Parkinson's disease is also associated with age and usually manifests itself after the age of 50, although the correlation with age is not as dramatic and ominous as for Alzheimer's disease. Both disorders are degenerative, involving a clear loss of neurons in the brain. The substantia nigra is the region affected by death of dopaminergic neurons in Parkinson's disease, while broader neuronal loss with cholinergic prevalence is observed in the brain of Alzheimer's disease patients.

Cerebral or spinal cord trauma and ischemia have come to be among the most common causes of death or impairment in recent years. The frequency of cerebral ischemic attack is apparently decreasing, but trauma is the major cause of death and impairment among young people. Epidemiological studies

S. Garattini (ed.), The Importance of Animal Experimentation for Safety and Biomedical Research, 57–69.

have shown that if the loss of years was taken into account instead of the number of the lost lifes, trauma would be causing social damage much greater than cancer and cardiovascular disorders, which mainly affect elderly people. Ischemia is an event secondary to neural trauma, and consequently therapeutic measures for both situations may be related. We still lack effective treatment for the acute phase of damage; in particular there is no hopeful treatment for spinal cord trauma yet. A better understanding of the primary and secondary damage to the nervous system following trauma and ischemia is required for developing appropriate therapies.

The peripheral nervous system is also affected by a variety of pathological conditions accompanied by axonal degeneration arising directly or indirectly as a correlate of a primary disease. In the case of trauma or exposure to toxic substances and as a result of unknown etiopathological agents in the case of amyotrophic lateral sclerosis (ALS), nerve degeneration is the primary damage. On the other hand degeneration of sensory and motor nerves as secondary events accompany metabolic disorders such as diabetes. Basic research has shown that peripheral nerves can regenerate and reinnervate the denervated organs.

Can we improve neuronal regeneration?

In this brief article we shall discuss present knowledge about degeneration and regeneration of neurons, and the necessary experimental models for new therapeutic strategies.

Mechanisms of axonal regeneration

Peripheral nerves and neuromuscular synapses have provided useful models for mechanisms of axonal degeneration and regeneration and for disappearance and reappearance of synaptic connection. Research into these problems may have begun with Abbott Felice Fontana, director of the Museum of Physics and Natural Sciences in Florence and personal physician to the Grand Duke of Tuscany. He described reconstruction of the lesion site suggesting that the damaged part had been 'reproduced' [1].

In more recent years, however, it has been shown that injured or dead neurons cannot be 'reproduced' by duplication of surviving ones. The transected axons or dendrites must regrow the lost processes [2]. Soon after nerve lesioning, Schwann cells undergo hypertrophy and begin phagocytosis of the degenerating axons; the nerve terminal degenerates within 8–14 hours [3]. The post-synaptic site is also altered; there is a major change in receptor distribution with an increase in the density of extra-synaptic ones so that the entire muscle fiber becomes sensitive to the neurotransmitter. This is termed supersensitivity and is a typical response of a target neuron to denervation [4].

The axon is an extension of the cell body lacking non-mitochondrial protein synthesis, that is exclusively located in the soma. Therefore all the material necessary for axonal maintenance and regrowth derives from the cell body and is transported along the entire axon as suggested many years ago by Ramon y Cajal [5].

Axonal transport is essential for axonal regeneration. It has been shown using a variety of *in vivo* experimental models that axonal transport involves at least five components and the most important part for regeneration seems related to slow transport that conveys the cytoskeleton.

All the cytoskeletal molecules are transported slowly in two waves, one moving at a rate of 0.25–2 mm/day (SCa) and the other at 2–5 mm/day (SCb) [6, 7]. The rate of axonal elongation is known to be 2–5 mm/day, corresponding to the higher rate of axonal transport, SCb [6, 7]. Axonal regeneration is preceded by a crucial process of sprouting by the injured axons, which a few days after injury, bud off a restricted number of processes. Only one or two sprouts per injured axon can cross the injured area of the nerve in case of crush injury, and in cases of sectioning the probability of success is much less [2].

Crossing the gap at the site of injury is one of the major problems for nerve microsurgery because of scar formation at the site of suture [8]. A variety of artificial protheses are now under development so that stretching and suture of the two stumps (proximal and distal) may be avoided. It is essential to establish a proper terrain favorable to axonal and vascular ingrowth. A plastic tube containing such material is sutured at its end to both stumps and the regenerating axons can be monitored growing from proximal to distal.

Another major problem for nerve regeneration is the rate of axonal elongation, that in humans is 1 mm/day at best and the length of certain nerves. If the lesion is in the upper portion of arms or legs, even the most effective nerve regeneration would take several months before reinnervating the most distal muscles, that consequently undergo severe atrophy [8]. There is an urgent need for developing nerve growth facilitating agents. The conditioning lesion paradigm offers some hope: if a nerve is lesioned a second time between two and three weeks after the primary nerve lesion the rate of nerve regeneration is augmented significantly [8]. This is an important therapeutic finding, and becomes even more important when the nerve lesion occurs in a patient with pathology that reduces the slow transport, such as diabetes [9].

What are the causes of axonal sprouting after injury?

What are the mechanisms leading to proper regrowth and reinnervation?

What is the sprouting capacity of a neuron?

These questions have been answered by a combination of *in vivo* and *in vitro* experiments.

The classic question, 'what is the cause of axonal sprouting', has been clearly answered by the simple and elegant experiments performed by Dennis Bray and colleagues [10, 11]. The growing neurite of a single chick sensory neuron in culture was amputated with a fine needle and the fates of the proximal and distal portions of the neurite were monitored. The amputated distal portion of the neurite collapsed and retracted, forming a bead in about 30 minutes.

Soon after a growth cone is formed from the bead, that grows at a rate similar to normal neurite growth in culture (40–100 μm/h). Formation of growth cones and growth can also be bipolar. The extension of the neurite is correlated to the decrease in size of the bead, suggesting that the bead material utilized for reformation of the neurite contains the bead. The final extension of the neurite is similar to the length of the amputated one. The proximal stump of the amputated neurite also retracts a little and forms a bead from which a new growth cone is formed and the neurite begins the elongation process again.

If neurons growing in culture are treated with colcemid that destroys microtubules, the cytoplasm collapses and a large number of spikes and growth cones are generated by the neurite [10, 11]. These data confirm the *in vivo* findings, suggesting that the potential for sprouting is present all along the axon, but is normally repressed, most likely by microtubules. This repression can be overcome by injury. In addition these data indicate that the cytoskeleton may be disorganized and reorganized locally, forming new axonal branches.

The growth cone is the tip of the regenerating axons and is apparently responsible for the direction of growth by recognizing the appropriate substrates of adhesion and elaborating a variety of environmental messages. By means of these abilities the growth cone must also be able to recognize the target for synapse reformation [2].

An example of such properties is provided by the following experiments *in vitro*. The growing tip of a chick sensory neuron was exposed to a gradient of nerve growth factor (NGF) diffusing out of a pipette. Within a few minutes the growth cone turned and then grew towards the pipette tip [12, 13]. These data showed that NGF, besides having trophic activity, also has tropic properties that are recognized by the growth cone.

As described above, axonal sprouting is defined as the necessary initial stage of outgrowth of new processes from injured or intact axons. Collateral sprouting was first described several decades ago. Muscles were partially denervated by transecting a portion of the nerve, and it was observed that the extent of denervation became gradually less and the muscle could eventually be completely reinnervated even if regeneration of the transected axons was inhibited. The recovery of muscle innervation was attributed to collateral outgrowth of the surviving intact axons still innervating the muscle [14–18].

Collateral sprouts can originate from nerve terminals, nodes of Ranvier, or the preterminal portion of the axon as illustrated in the figures 1–8. Sprouting occurs only intramuscularly, axons of extramuscular nerve trunks sprouting only after direct injury [19].

The limitation to the extent to which axons can sprout is a very important question for neuronal repair following injury. There is a limit to capacity for neuronal sprouting and reinnervation of denervated targets. Experimental results show that the field of innervation can be expanded up to 4–5 fold (Table 1). Sprouting capacity as represented by Index of Sprouting is greater when denervation is present to a larger extent. Aging might reduce sprouting

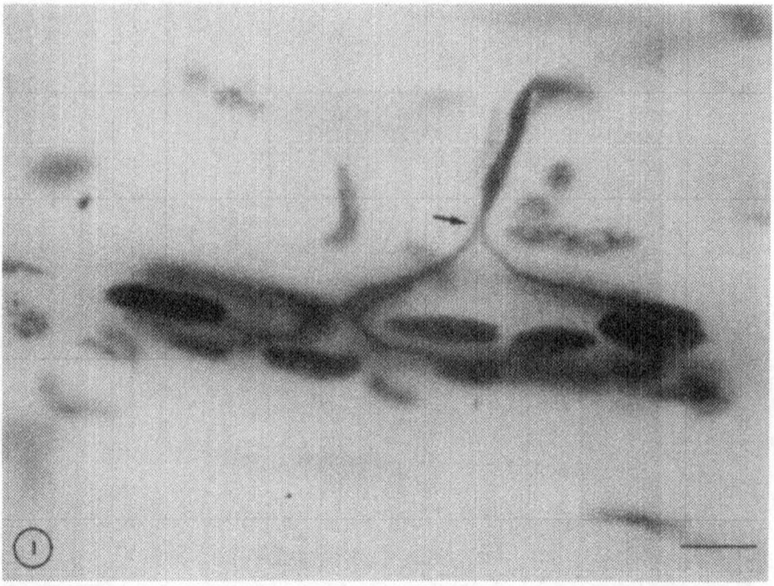

Fig. 1. Muscle end-plate. Silver impregnation and acetylcholinesterase. Reprinted from ref. 18, with permission of editor and authors.

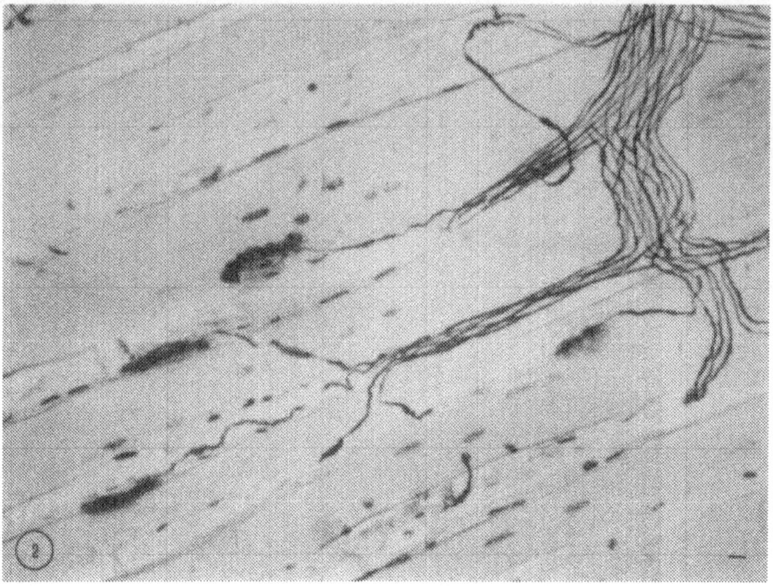

Fig. 2. Muscle innervation. Nerve trunks and single axons innervating end plates are shown. Reprinted from ref. 18 with permission.

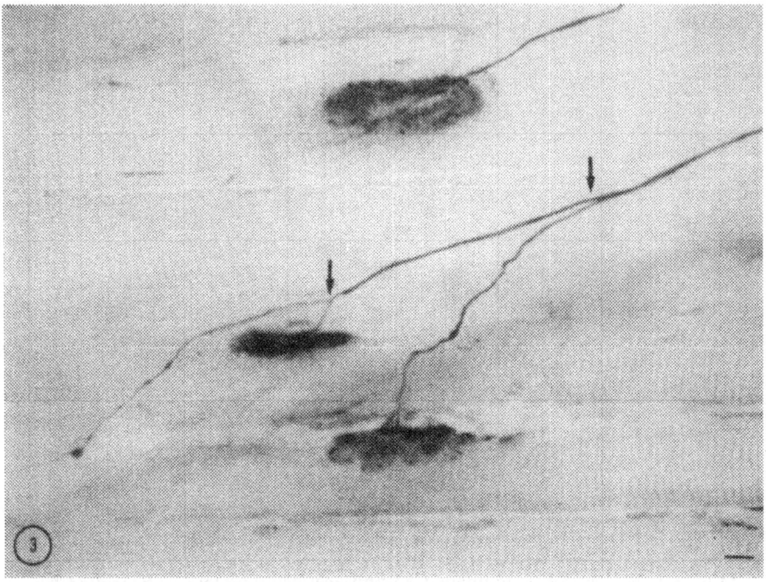

Fig. 3. Sprouting of a regenerating axon. Reprinted from ref. 18 with permission.

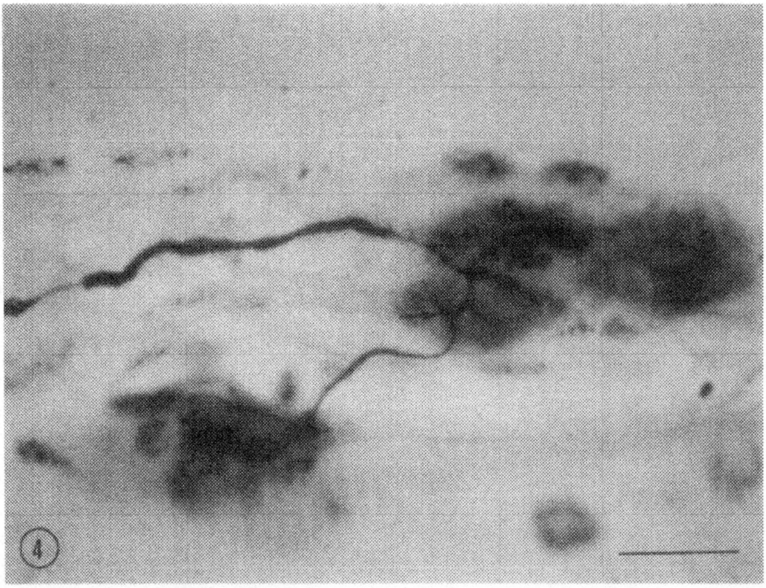

Fig. 4. Ultraterminal sprouting from an intact axon after partial denervation of a muscle. Reprinted from ref. 18 with permission.

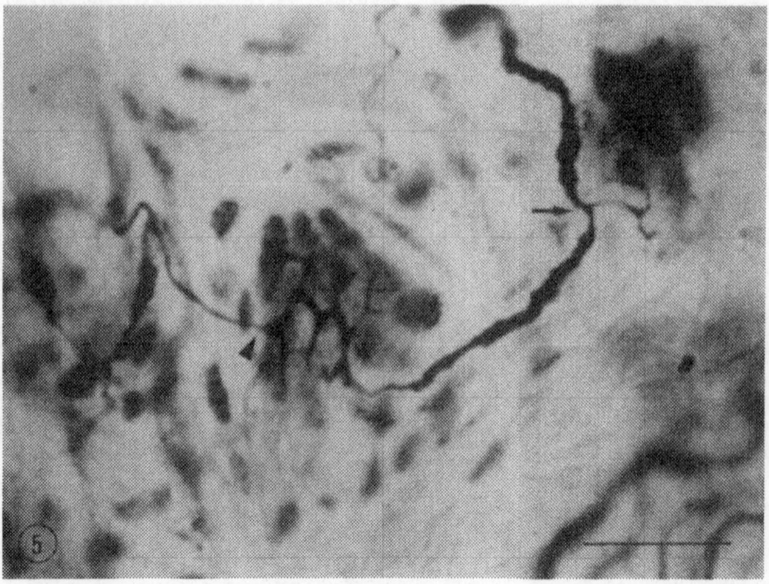

Fig. 5. Ultraterminal and nodal sprouting from an intact axon surviving partial denervation of a muscle. Reprinted from ref. 18 with permission.

capacity [20].

There may be several causes of sprouting in addition to injury with presynaptic activities such as axonal transport, excitability and transmitter release causes sprouting by the affected axons or by nearby intact ones [19]. Postsynaptic inactivity may cause sprouting of the innervating axons [19].

It was hypothesized that the denervated or inactive target could be releasing the substance responsible for stimulating sprouting. This suggestion was confirmed by *in vitro* findings of a neurite-promoting substance in extracts of denervated muscle fibers [21]. Subsequently, it has been shown that peripheral nerve injury causes NGF synthesis, probably by Schwann cells [22]. The process of synthesis is biphasic with an initial increase to peak production of mRNA for NGF within 10–12 hours post-lesion, followed by a significant drop at 24 hours. Then mRNA levels for NGF rise again. If the scietic nerve is dissected and placed *in vitro* mRNA production shows only the first phase [22]. In parallel to the mRNA for NGF the mRNA for its receptor also increases [22].

The production of trophic substances capable of enhancing neuronal survival and neurite production has also been detected in the cns by adding extracts of injured brain to cultures of neurons [23]. This production of neurotrophic substances can be correlated with sprouting in the dentate of the hippocampus following entorhinal cortex lesioning [23].

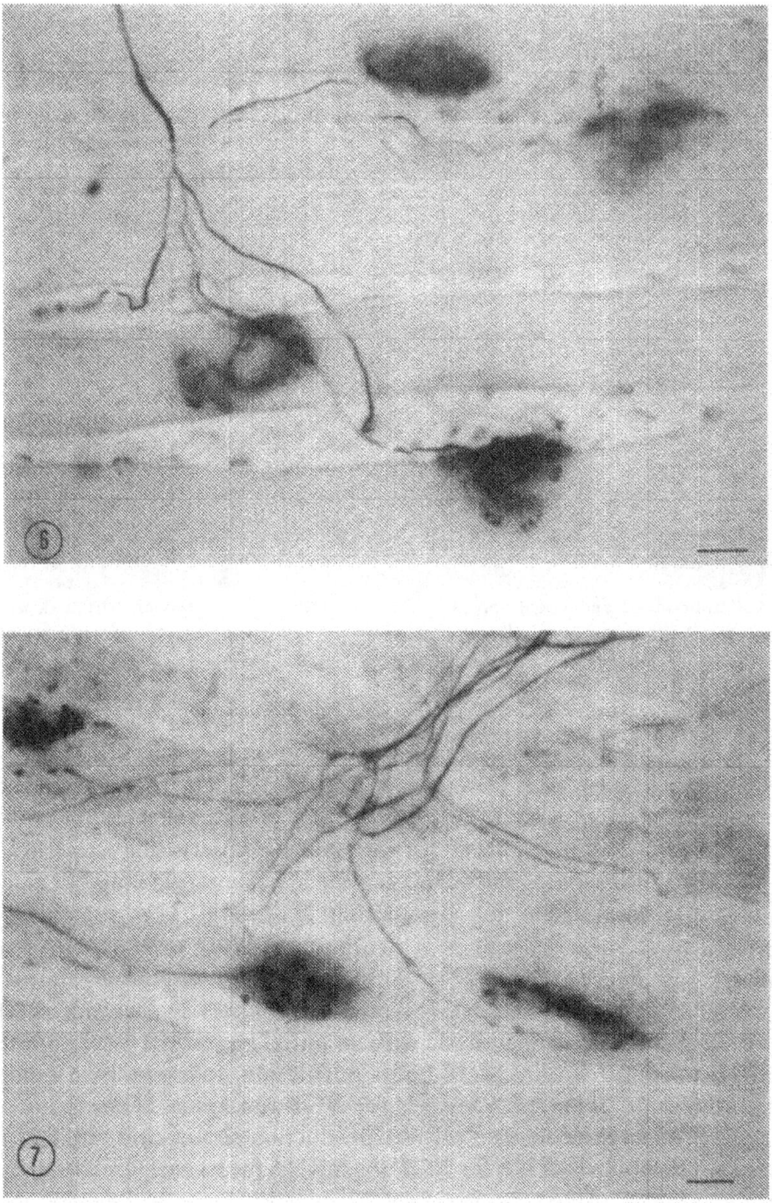

Figs 6–7. Multiple sprouting after partial denervation of a muscle. Reprinted from ref. 18 with permission.

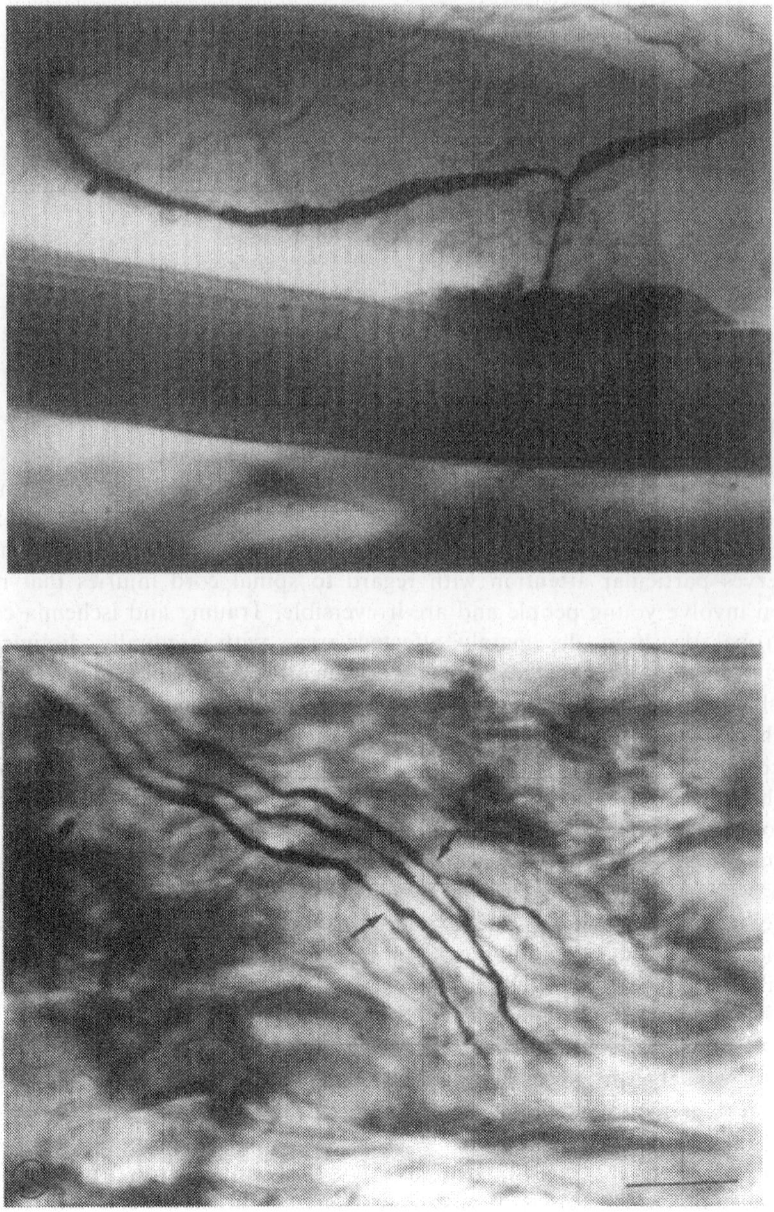

Figs 8–9. Nodal sprouting after partial denervation of a muscle. Reprinted from ref. 18 with permission.

Table 1. Index of sprouting

MU	IN	IR	IS
1	3.3	15.0	4.5
2	6.6	27.7	4.2
5	16.5	63.0	3.8
8	26.4	89.6	3.4

Reprinted from ref. [18], with permission of authors and editors.
MU = number of motor units remaining after partial denervation;
IN = percentage of the muscle normally innervated by that number of motor unit;
IR = percentage of the muscle innervated by the same number of motor units 30 days after partial denervation;
IS = Index of sprouting defined as the ratio between IR and IN.

Degenerative disorders of the central nervous system

As indicated in the introduction neural trauma and ischemia are forms of acute damage to the nervous system that still call for major scientific effort to overcome the lack of effective pharmacological treatments. The situation deserves particular attention with regard to spinal cord injuries that most often involve young people and are irreversible. Trauma and ischemia cause neuronal death in the mainly affected areas with gradually diminishing involvement of the adjacent areas. Identification of the various molecular mechanisms responsible for neural damage is associated with the development of therapeutic strategies to control those processes. If the deterioration could be controlled, neuronal survival would be improved and the neuronal networks in the affected areas could be spared with consequently less loss of function following the injury.

On account of the poor regenerative capacity of cns neurons, it is imperative that we aim for neuronal survival as a target. Recently three areas of research have been singled out as targets: lipid peroxidation, calcium influx as a cause of neuronal death, and excitatory amino acids. These lines of research have resulted in several potentially effective agents though extensive scientific and clinical evaluation is still necessary.

The acute damage affecting the lesion core starts within six hours after lesion, while the progressive damage affecting the periphery may take a week. The development of effective treatments must take in account this time course of neural damage.

Many degenerative neurological disorders show intraneuronal accumulation of neurofilaments. This is of particular relevance in the case of Alzheimer's disease, characterized by a complex mass of filaments named 'neurofibrillary tangles'. These filaments are quite different from normal neurofilaments. They react like amyloid corth green-red birefringence after Congo Red staining and have the structural appearance of tightly adherent pairs of helically wound intermediate filaments [24].

The second major alteration is the neuritic amyloid plaque. As reported above there is a specific cholinergic implication in Alzheimer's disease. Recent experimental results indicated that intracisternal infusion of NGF prevents cholinergic neuron death after axotomy, giving new hopes even for this disease [25].

A recent experimental breakthrough related to degenerative neurological disorders was obtained when it was established that in animals and man a synthetic substance mimicks the clinical syndrome of Parkinson's disease. The substance is known as MPTP (1-methyl-4-phenyl-1,2,3,6-tetrahydropyridine). Before this development studies were possible only on actual victims of the disease. Parkinson's complex symptoms are caused by degeneration of neurons in the substantia nigra, innervating the striatum, that coordinate and control complex movements. These neurons contain dopamine as neurotransmitter. In Parkinson's disease 80-90% of the dopaminergic neurons in the substantia nigra die, thus dopaminergic transmission in the striatum is greatly reduced even though the post-synaptic receptors are normal [26, 27]. Because dopamine receptors remain functional, pharmacological treatment aims at replenishing the striatal structures of dopamine to compensate its loss after neuronal death [28]. L-DOPA is used.

The ideal pharmacological treatment, however, should prevent neuronal death and stimulate regeneration and reinnervation, as explained earlier. The development of an MPTP animal model is supplying researchers with an appropriate tool for studying the disease progression and improving therapeutic strategies. Experimental studies are in fact showing that MPTP damage other areas affected too. Drugs can be tested for efficacy in MPTP animal models before being used in patients. This animal model is also providing suitable conditions for testing survival and effects of cell transplants in the nigra of striatum [29, 30].

Conclusions

In the past few years we have seen a blossoming of research dedicated to neuronal regeneration for a variety of reasons ranging from recent technological advances to the increasing social needs related to lengthening of the average human life. The latter point has created an urgent need for new therapeutic agents to improve neuronal regeneration and this achievement comes within reach through the appropriate use of experimental models both *in vivo* and *in vitro*. Naturally, *in vitro* systems can be utilized for screening agents effective on neuronal survival or regeneration but animal models are still necessary for establishing the efficacy of these substances in the appropriate conditions of neuronal degeneration, i.e. trauma, ischemia, various kinds of central and peripheral nervous system degeneration.

References

1. Fontana F (1781) Treatise on the venom of the viper; ... to which are annexed, observations on the primitive structure of the body. Different experiments on the reproduction of the nerves, 2 Vols. Murray, London.
2. Gorio A (1984) Sprouting and regeneration of peripheral nerve. In: E. Zagoren (Ed) *The Node of Ranvier*. Academic Press, New York, pp 353–388
3. Birks R, Katz B, Miledi R (1960) Physiological and structural changes at the amphibian myoneural junction in the course of nerve degeneration. *J Physiol* 150: 145–168
4. Axelsson J, Thesleff S (1959) A study of supersensitivity in denervated mammalian skeletal muscle. *J Physiol* 147: 178–193
5. Ramon y Cajal S (1928) Degeneration and regeneration of the nervous system. Oxford Press, London and New York, May R. M. (transl.) (1968), Hafner, New York
6. Black MM, Lasek RJ (1980) Slow components of axonal transport: two cytoskeletal networks. *J Cell Biology* 86: 616–623
7. Lasek RJ, McQuarrie, Wujek JR (1981) The central nervous system regeneration: Neuron and environment. In: A Gorio, H Millesi, Mingrino S (Eds), *Posttraumatic peripheral nerve regeneration: Experimental basis and clinical implications*. Raven Press, New York, pp 59–70
8. Gorio A, Millesi H, Mingrino S (Eds) *Posttraumatic peripheral nerve regeneration: Experimental bases and clinical implications*. Raven Press, New York (1981)
9. Vitadello M, Couraud JY, Hassig R, Gorio A, Di Giamberardino L (1983) Axonal transport of acetylcholinesterase in the diabetic mutant mouse. *Exp Neurol* 82: 143–147
10. Shaw G, Bray D (1977) Movement and extension of isolated growth cones. *Exp Cell Res* 104: 55–62
11. Bray D, Thomas C, Bray D (1978) Growth cone formation in cultures of sensory neurones. *Proc Natl Acad Sci* USA 75: 5226–5229
12. Gundersen RW, Barrett JN (1979) Neuronal chemotaxis: Chick dorsal root axons turn towards high concentrations of nerve growth factor. *Science* 206: 1079–1080
13. Gundersen RW, Barrett JN (1980) Characterization of the turning response of dorsal root neurites towards nerve growth factor. *J Cell Biol* 87: 546–554
14. Exner S (1885) Die Innervation des Kehlkopfes. *Sitzunsber Acad Wiss. Wien, Math-Naturwiss Kl* Abt 1, 89: 63–118
15. Hoffman H (1950) Local reinnervation in partially denervated muscle: A histophysiological study. *Ast J Exp Biol Med Sci* 28: 383–397
16. Van Harreveld A (1945) Reinnervation of denervated muscle fibers by adjacent functioning motor units. *Am J Physiol* 144: 447–493
17. Weiss P, Edds MV (1946) Spontaneous recovery of muscle following partial denervation. *Am J Physiol* 145: 587–607
18. Gorio A, Marini P, Zanoni R (1983) Muscle reinnervation. III. Motoneuron sprouting capacity, enhancement by exogenous gangliosides. *Neuroscience* 8: 417–429
19. Brown MC, Holland RL, Hopkins WG (1981) Motor nerve sprouting. *Annu Rev Neurosc* 4: 17–42.
20. Pestronk A, Drachman DB, Griffin JW (1980) Effects of aging on nerve sprouting and regeneration. *Exp Neurol* 70: 65–82
21. Henderson CE, Huchet M, Changeux J-P (1983) Denervation increases a neurite-promoting activity in extracts of skeletal muscle. *Nature* 302: 609–611
22. Heumann R, Lindholm D, Bandtlow CE, Meyer M, Radeke M, Misko T, Shooter E and Thoenen H (1988) Regulation of the synthesis of nerve growth factor and nerve growth factor receptor. In: A Gorio, JR Perez-Polo, J De Vellis, B Haber (Eds), *Neural development and regeneration. Cellular and molecular aspects.* Springer Verlag, Berlin, *ASI Series* Vol H 22: 273–283
23. Nieto-Sampedro M, Cotman C (1985) Growth factor induction and temporal order in central

nervous system repair. In: C Cotman (Ed), *Synaptic Plasticity*. Guilford Press, New York, 407–455

24. Wisniesky HM, Narang HK and Terry TD (1976) Neurofibrillary tangles of paired helical filaments. *J Neurol Sci* 27: 173–181
25. Gorio A, Perez-Polo J, De Vellis J, Haber B, Eds (1988) Neural development and regeneration. Cellular and molecular aspects. Springer Verlag, Berlin, *ASI Series* Vol H 22
26. Markey SP, Castagnoli N, Trevor AJ, Kopin IJ, Eds (1986) MPTP: A neurotoxin producing a Parkinsonian syndrome. Acad. Press, Orlando
27. Marsden CD, Fahn S, Eds (1982) Movement Disorders, *Butterworth Scientific*, London
28. Da Prada M, Keller HH, Pieri L, Kettler R and Hafely WE (1984) The pharmacology of Parkinson's disease: Basic aspects and recent advances. *Experientia* 40: 1165–1472
29. Bankiewicz KS, Oldfield EH, Chiueh CC, Doppman JL, Jacobiwitz, Kopin IJ (1986) Hemiparkinsonism in monkeys after unilateral internal carotid artery infusion of 1-methyl-4-phenyl-1,2,3,6-tetrahydropyridine (MPTP). *Life Sci* 39: 7–16
30. Backlund EO, Granberg PJO, Hamberger B, Knuttson E, Martesson A, Sedvall G, Seiger A, Olson L (1985) Transplantation of adrenal medullary tissue to striatum in parkinsonism. First clinical trials. *J Neurosurg* 62: 169–173

Endocrine glands, neuroendocrinology and animal experimentation

PAOLO PREZIOSI

Department of Pharmacology, Faculty of Medicine and Surgery, Catholic University of the Sacred Heart, Rome, Italy

The dawn of endocrinology and animal experimentation

Until the second half of the last century, certain ductless body organs delivering their secretory products externally (e.g. the adrenals, thymus, spleen and thyroid) were indicated as *ganglia sanguinea vasculosa* (vascular blood glands) [1] and were considered to be 'vestigial' structures. In fact, anatomists from the 16th to 19th centuries were able to discover many of these structures, but totally failed to imagine their ability to deliver the products of their secretion into the blood with consequent effects upon distant target tissues.

Vesalius (16th century) considered the pituitary with its infundibular process as a funnel that collected 'pituita' (phlegm, mucus) from the brain [2]; Willis (17th century) spoke of the pituitary as a structure collecting waste products from the brain. Littrius (same century) wrote that the pituitary was able to collect lymph from the brain, mix it with its own secretion (*cum succo partix rubellae proprio*) and release it in the circular veins (coronary sinus) (quoted by Pende, [1]). In 1563, Eustachi discovered the adrenals, but considered them as a gland pressing on the kidneys: *de glandulis qui renis incumbunt*.

The activity of endocrine glands was first perceived in the 17th and 18th centuries [1, 3]. The fact that something may be secreted by the testes, since their ablation led to eunuchism, caused Willis (1621–1675), quoted by Hoskins, [4] to write:

> 'the blood pours out something through the spermatic arteries to the genitals so also it receives as a recompense a certain ferment from the parts – to wit certain particles imbued with a seminal tincture are carried back to the blood... which make it vigorous and inspire into it a new and lively virtue'.

Ruysch (1638–1731) thought of the vascular blood glands as directly delivering secretory products to the blood. Hunter (1730) acknowledged secretory products flowing from the testes to the blood and subsequently to peripheral targets. Th. de Bordeaux (1775) talked about organs delivering specific substances able to display useful and stimulant actions to body preservation (quoted by Selye, [3]).

S. Garattini (ed.), The Importance of Animal Experimentation for Safety and Biomedical Research, 71–80.

Between 1830–44, Müller thought of some ductless glands (gefässknote) (adrenals, spleen, thymus, thyroid) as vascular blood glands with no contact with the external environment such as the other glands have (sie haben keine Beziehung auf ein Aüsseres wie die anderen Druse): i.e. he considered these glands as a separate entity able to display a plastic influence (einen plastischen Einfluss) on 'humours' circulating interiorly and delivered from there to the general circulation.

However, it was up to animal experimentation to provide a reliable demonstration that the 'vascular blood glands' produce something that can influence the whole body as well as specific characteristics.

In the 18th and 19th centuries, Hunter (1771) and Berthelit (1849) (quoted by Selye, [3] recognized the endocrine effects of the testes as preserving male traits in chickens by grafting the ablated testes to other body areas of the same animal.

It was not until 1856 that Brown-Séquard demonstrated, through ablation in animals, that the adrenal glands are essential to life. The first recognition of a possible delivery of a secretory product of these glands into the blood was by Vulpian (quoted by Collins, [5]) in 1856. He demonstrated that venous blood from the adrenals followed the same 'green' reaction with iron perchlorate as the medullary tissue of the adrenals: this was adrenaline, produced by the medullary chromaffin cells and delivered to the blood!

In 1855-56, Claude Bernard invented the term *sécrétion interne* as opposed to *sécrétion externe* of glands with excretory ducts, without yet recognizing the specialist internal secretion of the endocrine glands by the simple delivery of metabolic products (e.g. glucose from the liver) to the blood (quoted by Selye, [3]).

In 1856–57, Schiff found severe thyroid deficiency symptoms in animals after ablation of the gland. In 1869 Brown-Séquard was the first to give the name 'internal secretion glands' to what had previously been known as 'vascular blood glands'. In 1884, Horsley induced myxoedema like that found in humans by ablating the thyroid monkeys. In the same year, Schiff reported the

Table 1. Chronology of highlights in experimental endocrinology
(Reproduced, modified, from T.A. Thomas and E.T. Keenan [6]

1897	Von Mering and Minkowski pancreatomize dogs and produce characteristic symptoms of diabetes mellitus
1921	Banting and Best discover insulin
1925	Collip succeeds in using parathyroid extracts to elevate serum calcium
1929	Koch and associates use bull testes to produce comb growth in capons
1953	Pincus and co-workers describe the pituitary inhibitory effects of synthetic steroids in rabbits
1956	Rock, Garcia and Pincus demonstrate the ovulation-inhibiting actions of 'the pill' – norethynodrel – in women.

therapeutic value of replacement therapy (small grafts, thyroid extracts) in thyroid-ablated animals (quoted by Pende, [1]). Other highlights in experimental endocrinology are shown in Table 1.

General methods in endocrinology

Surgical extirpation of a gland, the demonstration that an extract of a gland can restore normal endocrine function, possibly followed by isolation of the pure hormone and, in some cases, synthesis of a congener of the hormone, are the classical methods that resulted - and may still do so - in the discovery of hormones or drugs acting through hormone-specific receptors [7]. In fact, ablation of glands and the ensuing symptomatology provide an understanding of the link between, for example, pancreas and diabetes, the adrenals and Addison's disease, or the pituitary and gonad dysfunctions. Moreover, glandular extracts (e.g. from the adrenals) and subsequently the purified hormones obtained from animal sources (e.g. insulin, parathyroid hormone) provided valuable treatments for once incurable human diseases.

Animal experimentation was - and still is - invaluable in providing suitable elements for ascertaining whether hormone secretion may be regulated by another hormone (e.g. corticotropin or cortisol), by neural influences (e.g. cholinergic stimulation of catecholamine release from the adrenal medulla), by concentration of a circular ion or metabolite (ionized calcium and parathyroid hormone glucose and glucagon), or all three kinds of regulation (as in the case of insulin-secreting beta cells of the pancreatic islets) [7].

Endocrine tests and the safety of new drugs

For the study of new drugs, a basic endocrine screen (a two-week test) has been considered advisable for about the last 25 years [8]. It may be performed on immature rats, the oral route being the administration of choice; anti-gonadotropic, androgenic (plus possible oestrogenic effects), anabolic, and corticosteroid-like activity are checked. Serum concentrations of the main hormone should also be assayed [9].

The importance of endocrine studies on animals for new drugs is clearly demonstrated by the recent history of etomidate (ETM). This is a phenyl imidazole [(R ±) ethyl 1-(phenyl-ethyl-1H-imidazole 5 carboxylate)] used as a short-lasting general anaesthetic suitable for induction, diagnostic procedures and minor surgery. Its advantages are rapid onset and short duration of action, less cardiovascular and respiratory depression than thiopental, the absence of histamine release and a possible cerebral protection against hypoxia [10]. In 1982, we found marked reduction of plasma corticosterone after narcotic doses of ETM (2.5–5 mg/kg) in rats, under both basal and surgical stress conditions, with a good dose/time/effect ratio (Table 2) [11].

Table 2. Effect of pretreatment with i.v. etomidate on plasma corticosterone concentrations in resting conditions and after laparotomy
(Reproduced from Preziosi and Vacca, 1982)

Treatment mg/kg	Lapa-rotomy	Plasma corticosterone (μg/dl) at the following times (in min)			
		4	30	60	360
Saline (2 ml/kg)	—	20.1 ± 1.1	20.0 ± 1.3	18.7 ± 2.6	17.1 ± 1.4
Etomidate 2.5	—		15.2 ± 0.9[a]	15.8 ± 1.3	17.3 ± 1.7
Etomidate 5	—	20.2 ± 1.2	6.9 ± 0.7[a]	9.5 ± 1.3[a]	17.2 ± 1.4
Saline (2 ml/kg)	yes	31.5 ± 1.7[a]	46.9 ± 2.5[a]	47.0 ± 2.6[a]	31.7 ± 1.5[a]
Etomidate 5	yes	22.8 ± 1.1[b]	18.0 ± 0.9[b]	19.7 ± 1.0[b]	22.7 ± 0.6[b]

* Samples were taken 2 min after the beginning of stress and 4–30–60–360 min from the injection of etomidate. These doses of etomidate employed provoked a narcosis lasting about 10 min. For each experimental group at least 8 animals were used.
[a] $P < 0.01$ with respect to saline-injected unstressed rats.
[b] $P < 0.01$ with respect to saline-injected stressed rats.

Table 3. Case fatality rates by types of sedation

ISS	Opiates and benzodiazepines	Opiates and etomidate	P
All patients	12/47 (25%)	18/26 (69%)	<0.0005
10–20	1/16 (6%)	4/8 (50%)	<0.05
21–30	4/11 (36%)	7/9 (77%)	NS
>30	7/20 (35%)	9/9 (100%)	<0.002

(Reproduced from Ledingham and Watt [12]).

Some time later, Ledingham and Watt [12] reported from Glasgow that the cause of elevated case fatality among seriously-injured patients in their unit compared with previous years might be related to the use of ETM by infusion instead of benzodiazepine in association with opiates in long-term sedation regimens (Table 3).

The finding that blood cortisol levels were extremely low in patients receiving prolonged infusions of ETM under clinical conditions identical to those of others who were not given the compound [13], and the observation that administration of cortisol reduced mortality in this group of patients [14] led to the awareness that ETM may interfere with adrenocortical function in humans [12] as had previously been shown in rats by us for (±) and (–) etomidate [10]. At the same time it was shown again in rats that (±) or (–) etomidate blocked the stimulatory effect of tetracosactrin (cosyntropin, ACTH 1–2n) on the adrenal cortex [15]. Had the drug-induced blockade of the adrenals under stress, as seen in rats, served as an adequate warning for humans, subsequent unfortunate clinical events might never have happened.

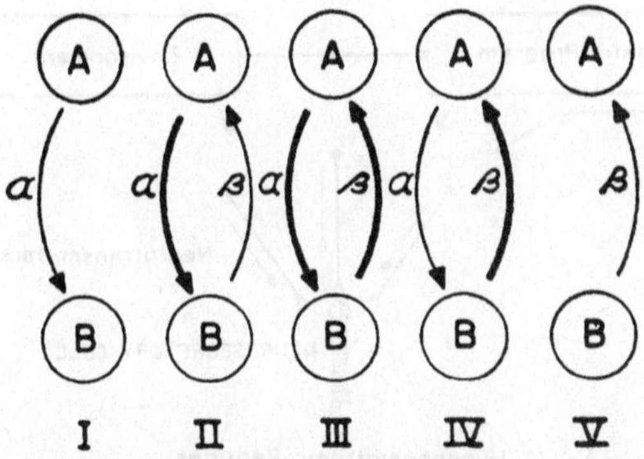

Fig. 1. Different phases of hormonal feedback as described in the text. Hormone concentration in the circulating blood is indicated by the thickness of the arrows. (Reproduced from Scharrer and Scharrer [16]).

Neuroendocrinology and animal experimentation

Neuroendocrinology may be considered to have begun with the observations by Wharton (1614–1673) (quoted by Pende, [1]) concerning the adrenals *plus quam probabile est nervum aliquid adverre vel auferre ab isce glandulis* (it is most probable that a nerve brings to and carries away something from these glands) and by Morgagni (1733) concerning the absence of the adrenal cortex in anencephalics. Neuroendrocrinology [2] may be characterized by balanced circuits formed by neural inputs controlling hypothalamic peptidergic cells, hormone-secreting structures (e.g. the anterior pituitary) and lastly target-stimulated hormones modulating the primary signal (feedback), all highly valuable examples of integrated systems [16] that cannot at present be studied outside the intact animal.

A simple feedback system is shown in Fig. 1. Organ A releases hormone α that stimulates endocrine organ B to produce and release hormone β. Increasing blood concentrations of the hormone begin to exert an inhibiting effect on organ A. As a result, the latter reduces its output and eventually ceases to release hormone α. Thus hormone β not only performs its own function, whatever that may be, but also regulates its own production by its inhibitory effect on organ A [16].

Endocrine organs, though, cannot by themselves make decisions on the basis of information other than the type just described. Thus, the feedback cycle must be open to allow the entry of messages that may change the existing pattern. For example, an important source of stimuli for the release of hormones controlling reproductive functions resides in the olfactory apparatus. The secretion of prolactin in mated female mice is depressed by olfactory stimuli caused by the presence of strange males resulting in blocking of pregnancy. This does not occur in females made anosmic through sectioning of the olfactory nerves [17]. The nerve centres in which the hormonal and nervous pathways

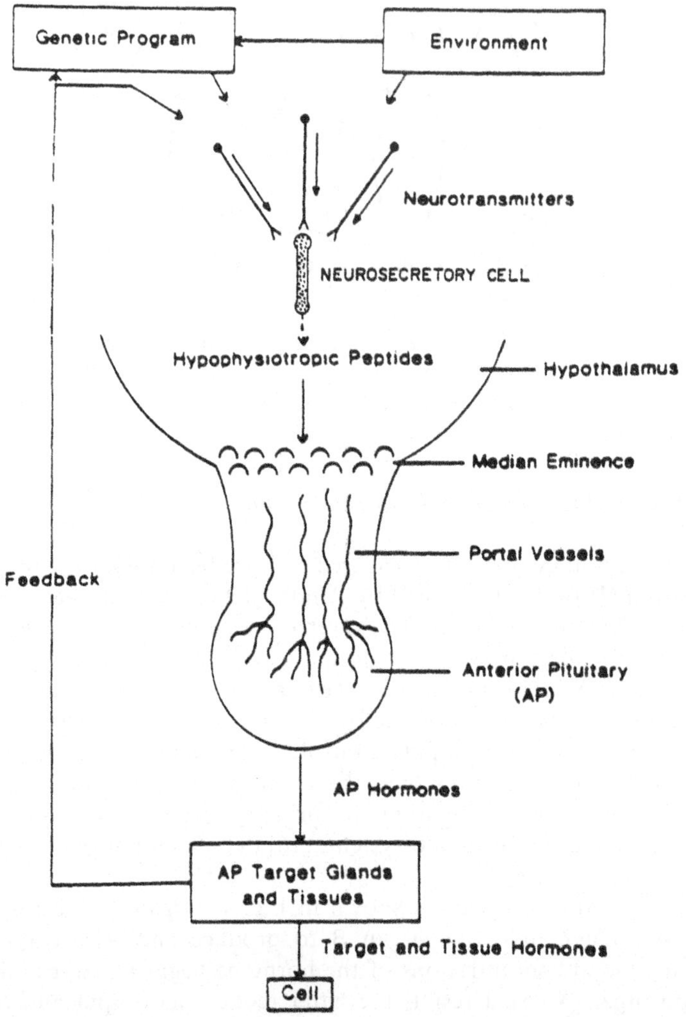

Fig. 2. Diagram illustrating neuroendocrine reactions and pathways by which the genome and environmental agents help control endocrine functions. The hypothalamus contains neurotransmitters which can modify the release of hypophysiotropic hormones that enter the portal vessels which originate in the median eminence (the 'final common pathway' between the brain and anterior pituitary [AP]). The hormones of the AP regulate secretion of hormones by the thyroid (T3,T4) gonads (estrogen, progesterone, testosterone, etc.), and adrenals (gluco- and mineral corticoids, sex hormones), and modify hormone secretion by the pancreas (insulin, glucagon), liver (somatomedins), gastrointestinal tract, and other tissues (brain, thymus, heart, etc.). Some AP hormones can also act directly on non-hormone secreting tissues to influence their growth and function. Hormones from the target glands and other tissues deef back on the hypothalamus to help control secretion of neurotransmitters and hypophysiotropic hormones. Hormones can also directly interact with the genome to modify its function. (Reproduced, modified, from Meites *et al.* [20]).

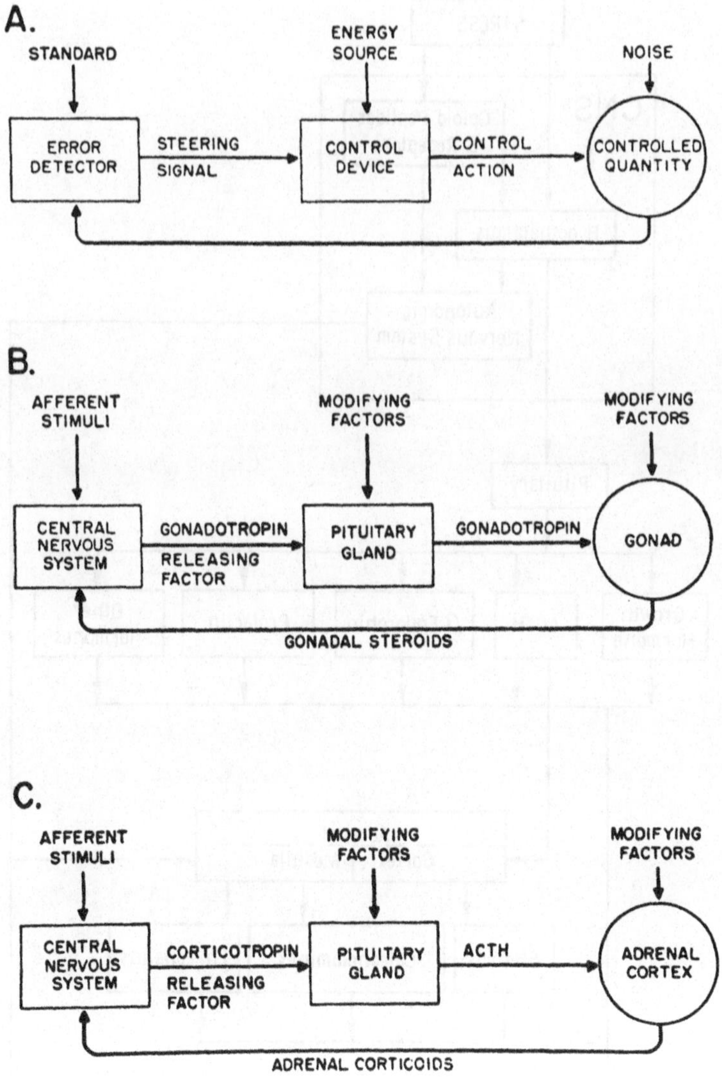

Fig. 3. Comparison of concepts of feedback systems in physics and neuroendocrinology. (A) Feedback system as of a thermostat controlling a furnace; (B) analogous hormonal feedback system controlling gonadal functions; (C) corresponding control system of the adrenal cortex. (Reproduced from Scharrer and Scharrer [16]).

terminate may also be affected by factors such as the concentration of salt or sugar in the blood, its temperature and other variables, such as the supraoptic nucleus in the mammalian hypothalamus to serve as osmoreceptors. For many integrated functions controlled by the hypophyseal hormone and their target areas (Fig. 2) the integration can take place only in the central nervous system.

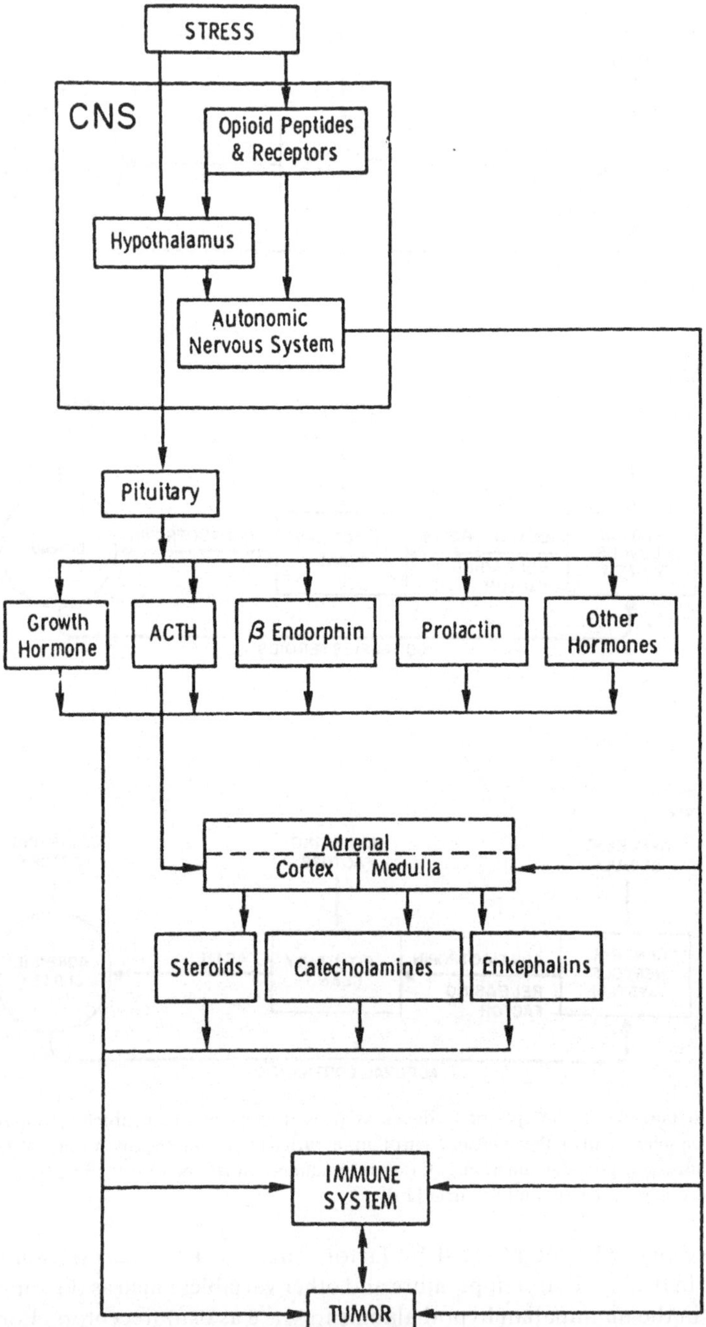

Fig. 4. Summary of neural and neurohumoral mechanisms by which stress might affect the immune system and tumours. (Reproduced, modified, from Shavit *et al.* [25]).

Unique neurosecretory cells, linked to nerve terminals, release the hypophysiotropic hormone. Afferent stimuli reach these cells and the resulting relationship resembles the concept of feedback as it is used in physics (Fig. 3).

Adrenal and ovarian function, the control of water and electrolytes are meaningful examples. How would it have been possible to detect such integrated systems and functions without animal experimentation? Animal experimentation has provided useful information concerning particular functions of the CNS which were found to be hormone-controlled. For example, the squatting position assumed up to the 19th week by the male dog when urinating, which subsequently changes to the typical male position of lifting a leg, may be abolished by castration, restored by androsterone, and its appearance advanced to the 8th week [9] by the same treatment. This means that the neural pattern is ready and hormones bring it to maturation.

The endocrine effects of the majority of psycho- and neural-active drugs are due to their suprahypophyseal interference. These drugs interact with receptors on nerve terminals approaching the hypothalamic peptidergic (neurosecretory) cells or located on the neurosecretory cells themselves [20] (Fig. 2). It should be remembered that decreased libido, impotence and amenorrhea observed after high-dose neuroleptic treatments could be due not only to increased prolactin release consequent on hypophyseal lactotroph blockade, but also to antidopaminergic and anti-adrenoceptor actions in the hypothalamus, with ensuing GnRH and hence reduced FSH and LH release [21]. Opioids [21] release prolactin and ACTH by acting on nerve circuits travelling to the hypothalamic peptidergic cells [22–24].

Any drug interference at any part of the neuroendocrine circuits (e.g. hormone binding to selected plasma proteins) may disrupt the whole homeostatic system.

More recently, neuroendocrine circuits were found to be able to interact with the immune system. Thus stress (Fig. 4) could strongly influence this system and consequently tumour growth [25].

Claude Bérnard now appears to have been really enlightened when he wrote [26]:

Quand on réunit des elements physiologiques, on voit apparaître des propriétés qui n'étaient pas appréciables dans ces éléments séparés (when physiological elements are assembled, properties not perceivable in the separate physiological elements may appear).

Animal experimentation has been and remains invaluable for the study of this fundamental integrated system.

References

1. Pende N (19xx) *Endocrinologia, Patologia e Clinica degli organi a secrezione interna*, Soc. Ed. Libraria, Milano, V Ediz.
2. Preziosi P (1983) Neuroendocrinologie et Neuroendocrinopharmacothérapie *Méd Hyg* 41:

771-772
3. Selye H (1952) *Trattato di endocrinologia*, Casa Editrice Ambrosiana, Milano
4. Hoskins RG (1941) *Endocrinology* W.W. Norton and Co Inc., p. 16
5. Collins R (1938) *Les hormones*, Ed. Albin Michel, Paris, p. 14
6. Thomas JA, Keenan E (1986) *Principles of endocrine pharmacology*, Plenum Med. Book Co., New York
7. Bourne HR (1987) Introduction to endocrine pharmacology. In: Katzung BG *Basic and clinical pharmacology*, 3rd ed., Appleton and Lange, Norwalk, pp. 414–423.
8. Zbinden G (1963) Experimental and clinical aspects of drug toxicity, *Adv Pharmacol* 2: 1, Academic Press
9. Katzung BG, Berkowitz B (1987) Basic and clinical evaluation of new drugs. In: Katzung BG *Basic and clinical pharmacology*, 3rd ed., Appleton and Lange, Norwalk, pp. 44–52.
10. Preziosi P, Vacca M (1988) Adrenocortical suppression and other endocrine effects of etomidate, *Life Sci* 42: 477–489
11. Preziosi P, Vacca M (1982) Etomidate and corticotrophic axis, *Arch Int Pharmacodyn Ther* 256: 308–310
12. Ledingham I, MCA, Watt I (1983) Influence of sedation on mortality in critically ill multiple trauma patients, *Lancet* I: 1270
13. Ledingham I, MCA, Finlay WEJ, Watt I, Mckee JI (1983) Etomidate and adrenocortical function, *Lancet* I: 1434
14. Mckee JI, Finlay WEJ (1983) Cortisol replacement in severely stressed patients, *Lancet* I: 484
15. Preziosi P (1983) Etomidate, sedatives and neuroendocrine changes, *Lancet* II: 276
16. Scharrer E, Scharrer B (1963) Neuroendocrinology, Columbia University Press
17. Parkes AS, Bruce HM (1961) Olfactory stimuli in mammalian reproduction, *Science* 134: 1049–1054
18. Verney EB, The antidiuretic hormone and the factors which determine its release, *Proc Roy Soc London* B135: 25–106
19. Berg IA, Development of behaviour: the micturition pattern in the dog, *J Expl Psychol* 34: 343-368.
20. Meites J, Goya R, Takahashi S (1987) Why the neuroendocrine system is important in aging processes, *Exp Gerontology* 22: 1–15
21. Johnstone EC, Ferrier IN (1980) Neuroendocrine markers of CNS drug effects, *Br J Clin Pharmacol* 10: 5–21
22. Meites J, Bruni JF, Van Vugt DA, Smith AF (1979) Relation of endogenous opioid peptides and morphine to neuroendocrine functions, *Life Sci* 24: 1325–1336
23. Morley JE (1981) The endocrinology of opiates and opioid peptides, *Metabolism* 30: 195-209
24. Stansfield SC, Knight PG, Howles CM, Cunningham FG (1988) Endogenous opioid peptide modulation of LH secretion in the ewe lambs: possible involvement of 5-hydroxytryptamine, *J Endocrinol* 116: 403–411
25. Shavit Y, Terman GW, Martin FC, Lewis JW, Liebeskind JC, Gale RP (1985) Stress, opioid peptides, the immune system and cancer, *J Immunol* 135: 834–837
26. Bernard C (1865) Introduction à l'étude de la médecine expérimentale, Paris, J.B. Baillière et Fils

Laboratory animals and cardiovascular pathology: Means for better use

JEAN SASSARD
Department of Physiology and Clinical Pharmacology UA CNRS 606, College of Pharmacy, Lyon, France

Introduction

The last few years have been marked by considerable progress in research strategy for new pharmacologically active molecules. From the simple systematic observation of effects which are not looked for *a priori* a much more mechanistic approach has been developed. This was made possible by the development of physiological and pathophysiological knowledge and by discoveries related to the molecular mechanism of action of enzymes, hormones and/or neurotransmitters implicated in physiological or pathological processes.

Cardiovascular pathology in developed countries is the greatest cause of disease and mortality and in this field one of the best examples of this molecular approach is provided by the synthesis of inhibitors of the angiotensin conversion enzyme. Interest in this enzyme derives from knowledge regarding the role of the angiotensin renin system in the control of blood pressure and in the pathophysiology of some forms of hypertension. The synthesis of inhibitors active by the oral route was made possible by determining the configuration of the active enzyme site, and the overall results led to the development of a remarkable new class of therapeutic drugs.

If these data are extrapolated, it may be thought that it would now suffice to identify a molecular target implicated in a pathological process, to define its physicochemical characteristics and to synthesise pharmacological modulators and verify their action, *in vitro*, to obtain a medicament. In fact, this is not the case. If the example of the angiotensin renin system inhibitor is examined, it will be noted that these relied on *in vivo* investigations which were the only way of: 1) demonstrating the beneficial action of enzyme conversion inhibitors on cardiac insufficiency, their very particular effect on left ventricular hypertrophy and on that of hypertensive arterial walls; 2) discovering its deleterious effects on renal function already altered by the hypertensive process; 3) demonstrating the toxicity of direct renin inhibitors.

Thus, I need hardly stress the evident necessity of having recourse to animal experimentation in the investigation of new medicaments and shall focus, in this exposé, on the following two points:

S. Garattini (ed.), The Importance of Animal Experimentation for Safety and Biomedical Research, 81–87.

- the complexity of cardiovascular functions and thus of their pathology. This makes it impossible now, and for some time to come, to set up any efficient model and must shed doubt on any over-simplification of the problem. This must lead to a very active search for more pertinent experimental models;
- the need, in view of the above point, to make better use of the data provided by animal experimentation through better scheduling of work and improvement in the number and quality of the variables gathered.

The need for new animal models

From the physiological point of view, the cardiovascular system is distinguished by its multi-factored nature. It has a multiplicity of structures – heart, vessels, and blood cells; a multiplicity of regulation factors – central nervous system, autonomous nervous system, hormones, enzymes. Moreover, as is shown in Fig. 1, each of these sub-systems comprises various participants which exchange considerable 'local' information amongst themselves.

As a consequence of this complexity, the physiopathology of cardiovascular disorders often remains partially or totally unknown. This is the case in particular of the two most frequent disorders – arterial hypertension and atherosclerosis. Human arterial hypertension is of undefined etiology in 90% of the cases. It is termed 'essential' and all that is known is that it responds to a genetic determinism. Atherosclerosis calls into play at least four cell types in the constitution of arterial plaque: endothelial cells, platelets, smooth muscle cells and macrophages. Epidemiological investigations have clearly shown that its development depends on a lipid overload, although the mechanisms are still not understood. Finally, in both cases, hypertension and

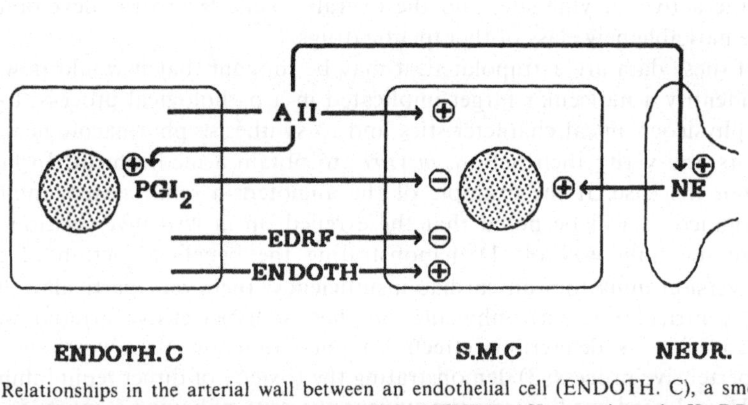

Fig. 1. Relationships in the arterial wall between an endothelial cell (ENDOTH. C), a smooth muscle cell (SMC) and a sympathetic nerve ending (NEUR.). AII = angiotensin II; PGI2 = prostacyclin; EDRT = endothelium derived relaxing factor; ENDOTH = endothelium; NE = noradrenalin.

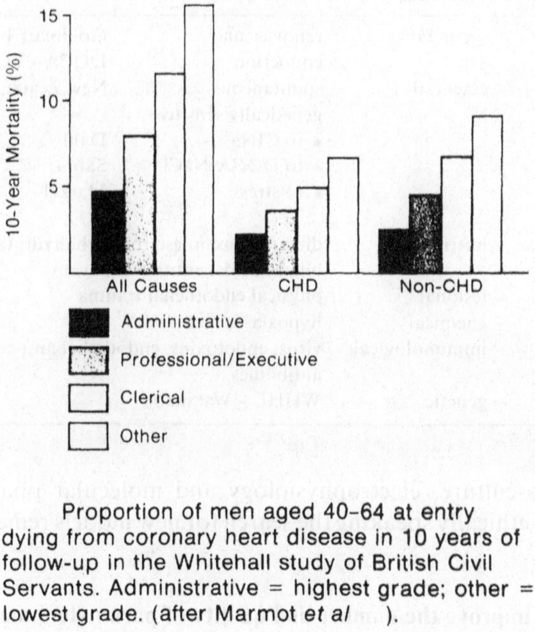

Fig. 2. Influence of social status on total mortality (all causes), coronary (CHD) and non-coronary (non-CHD).

atherosclerosis, expression of the disease depends on complex environmental factors, as is shown in Fig. 2 [1].

From here, any therapeutic advance implies the development of more appropriate animal models, which are indispensable for several reasons:

1. To understand more fully the pathophysiological mechanisms and identify new molecular targets likely to respond to pharmacological modulation. In this regard, the development of molecular biology provides great hope, for all diseases with a genetically determined nature. Thus, the USA gives pride of place to models developed in the mouse, whose genome is well known, in the aim of gaining a better understanding of the disorders observed.
2. To assess the efficacy of new molecules more precisely before administering them to humans.

The fact that there are so many models (cf. Table 1) for hypertension and atherosclerosis indicates that none of them is completely satisfactory. Thus experiments using several models must always be done requiring a larger number of laboratory animals. Identical observations can be made for the other severe cardiovascular pathologies: coronary ischemia, cerebral ischemia, cardiac insufficiency and rhythm disorders.

In conclusion, despite the progress made in biochemistry, cell culture and

Table 1. Principal animal models for arterial hypertension and atherosclerosis

Hypertension	– secondary	: renovascular	Goldblatt 1 or 2 kidneys
		endocrine	DOCA-CaCl
	– essential	: spontaneous	New Zealand, Japan, France, Italy
		genetically sensitive	
		• to ClNa	Dahl
		• to DOCA-NaCl	Sabra
		• to stress	Markel
Atherosclerosis	– nutritional	diets rich in cholesterol, carbohydrates and biliary acids, antithyroid agents	
	– lesional	physical endothelial trauma	
	– chemical	hypoxia	
	– immunological	virus, endotoxins, endothelial anti-cell antibodies...	
	– genetic	WHHL – Watanabe	

even cell co-culture, electrophysiology and molecular pharmacology, scientifically and ethically speaking the search for new models remains indispensable.

The need to improve the number and quality of parameters measured in the animal

I shall take the example of arterial pressure, since it is very demonstrative. The basic data are as follows:

- in the animal, as in the human, arterial pressure is a parameter which very rapidly varies with time and is greatly influenced by stress and physical and mental activity;
- although variable, arterial pressure is nonetheless subject to a multitude of reflex regulations;
- finally, it is technically difficult to determine and only direct, surgical methods can provide reference values.

Under these conditions, two broad sets of techniques are used: 1) direct surgical measurement of pressure in the anesthetised animal with all this implies in the way of stress and modification of reflex regulation; 2) indirect, non-surgical measurement in the conscious but usually excited animal. In this case the interference of the anesthesia is absent, but only a restricted quantity of data can be recorded, chronologically rather distanced.

Given the evidence, these methodological limitations have not prevented the discovery of extremely active molecules, but this has been achieved at the price of using large groups of experimental animals, and results were sometimes not very predictive of what was later to be observed in humans.

For some years, various groups have been developing techniques for continuously recording arterial pressure (AP) directly in the small conscious unrestrained animal, that is, without the interference of anesthesia and stress.

In this particular case [3] a data processing system was added for digital processing of the blood pressure curve and data storage with a view to subsequent analysis. Under these conditions, values for systolic, diastolic and mean arterial pressure, heart rate (HR), an index of cardiac flow and arterial relaxation during diastole were obtained for each heart beat. From there, moreover, two peripheral flows could be measured by implanted Doppler micro-probes, with one direct measurement of sympathetic nervous activity.

Since then, this technique, which requires a very sophisticated data processing system, has permitted more than 400,000 values of AP or HR per 24 hours to be obtained in the conscious unrestrained and unstressed rat, that is, under excellent conditions. It follows that significant observations can be made with small groups of animals, while the conventional indirect measurement methods either required a large number of experimental subjects, or were made difficult by the major interferences inherent in stress and the anesthesia.

Thus, it is possible to know not only the level of blood pressure but also:

1. Its spontaneous variability expressed by the standard deviation of values collected over a period of time. This is an important parameter, since Parati [4] demonstrated that for a given pressure level increased variability raises the cardiovascular risk;
2. Whether anesthesia leads to erroneous assessment of the severity and even the mechanism of action of an antihypertensive agent. It was in this manner that it was observed that in the anesthetised rat, that is, in a state of sympathetic hyperactivity, an agonist of adrenergic alpha2 receptors such as clonidine, markedly lowered AP and HR, regardless of whether it was administered *i.v.* or by the intra-cerebroventricular route. This very classical observation is at the basis of the concept of the antihypertensive agent with central action, of which clonidine is the prototype. Nonetheless, if this study is repeated in the unrestrained conscious rat, that is, with basal orthosympathetic activity, *i.v.* clonidine is much less effective than in the anesthetised rat, and is completely ineffective when injected intra-cerebroventricularly. These data confirm that clonidine lowers AP by way of a decrease in sympathetic activity but reveals that, under these basic conditions, analogous to those encountered in the ambulatory patient, the central component of its action seems to be very limited;
3. The determination, using a small number of animals, of the intensity and kinetics of the effects of a new molecule and the prediction, with adequate reliability, of what it will do in humans. This was the case in our experiment using new calcium blockers, only one of which was worth developing but needs further galenical work in order to limit the aggressiveness of its action and prolong its duration [5]. Likewise, for a new conversion enzyme inhibitor, it was quickly apparent that a single daily dose would be largely sufficient [6].
4. Finally, recently, the possibility of quantifying the variability of arterial pressure has led to a demonstration that prolonged chemical sympathectomy did not modify mean arterial pressure but increased its variability in the

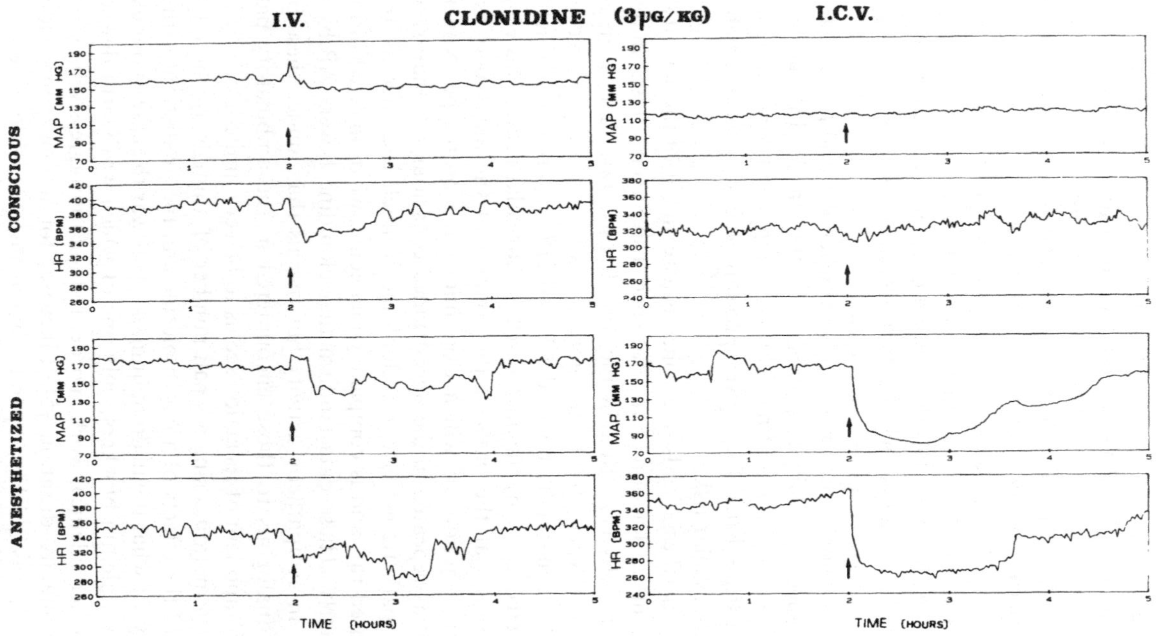

Fig. 3. Influence of anesthesia with pentobarbital on the cardiovascular effects of clonidine administered intravenously (*i.v.*) or intracerebroventricularly (*i.c.v.*); mean arterial pressure (MAP); heart rate (HR).

rat. This has a physiological consequence. The sympathetic system controls the variability of pressure by lowering it through the reflexes which call it into play, but does not affect its mean level which is determined by other factors, the first of which is the angiotensin-renin system. This observation may have therapeutic consequences which remain to be assessed with precision.

Thus, a purely methodological improvement makes the results obtained in the animal and more considerably reduces the number of experiments required to obtain any given information.

In conclusion, it would appear that in a field as complex as cardiovascular pathology, animal experimentation is and will remain absolutely indispensable for some time to come. Nonetheless, it is methodologically possible and ethically imperative to limit its extension by the development of new models and improvement in the number and quality of the data collected in the animal.

References

1. Marmot MG, Shipley MJ and Rose G (1984) Inequalities in death – specific explanation of a general pattern? *Lancet* 1: 1003–1006.
2. Cerutti C, Paultre CZ, Barrès C and Sassard J (1985) Computer analysis of intraarterially recorded blood pressure in conscious unrestrained rats. *J Pharmacol Methods* 13: 249–260.
3. Parati G, Pomidossi G, Albini F, Malaspina D and Mancia G (1987) Relationship of 24-hour blood pressure mean and variability to severity of target-organ damage in hypertension. *J Hypertension* 5: 93–98
4. Barrès C, Cerutti C, Morin B and Sassard J (1988) Cardiovascular effects of two new calcium antagonists PY 108-068 and PN 200-110, in conscious spontaneously hypertensive rats. *Br J Pharm* 93: 176–184
5. Barrès C, Cerutti C, Paultre CZ and Sassard J (1986) Antihypertensive effects of S9490-3, a new converting enzyme inhibitor in the conscious spontaneously hypertensive rat. *Clin Sci* 70: 167–175

The importance of animal models for hypertension research

D. GANTEN, K. LINDPAINTNER, Th. UNGER and J. MULLINS
German Institute for High Blood Pressure Research and Department of Pharmacology, University of Heidelberg, Heidelberg, FRG

Summary

Hypertension represents one of the most serious public health problems, both in terms of the number of people affected or at risk and in view of its long-term sequelae which are a major cause of morbidity and mortality in our societies. Despite continued research efforts, primary hypertension, which accounts for the vast majority of cases, remains poorly understood and is thus amenable only to palliative treatments. Based on epidemiological and experimental data, however, one can be fairly certain that primary hypertension is a genetically transmitted, inheritable disease. Studies directed at clinical problems such as hypertension are limited by the fact that neither *in vitro* and *in vivo* test systems nor computer simulation are able to provide a precise experimental counterpart for a human disease. Meaningful generalizations from experimental models to human disease are difficult. Evidence suggests, however, that several models of experimental hypertension, in particular the genetically hypertensive rat, share a number of important features with primary hypertension in humans. Thus, use of these models in conjunction with proper scientific questions and appropriate research methodology has improved our understanding of the disease and the possibilities for its treatment and prevention.

The introduction of transgenic rats into hypertension research represents a powerful new approach to the study of this disease and is expected to lead to significant advances in its understanding. To be put to use appropriately and productively, this technique calls for a concerted effort involving scientists working in different areas and on different aspects of hypertension.

Introduction

High blood pressure is one of the major medical problems in developed countries because of its high incidence (15–10%) and its serious long-term complications. End-organ damage leading to ischemic heart disease, cerebro-

S. Garattini (ed.), The Importance of Animal Experimentation for Safety and Biomedical Research, 89–96.

vascular accidents, chronic renal failure, and peripheral vascular disease all are important contributors to overall morbidity and mortality. Few public health issues represent a greater challenge to researchers and clinicians alike. In a small percentage of cases, hypertension develops as a secondary complication of another, treatable disorder, e.g. renal artery stenosis. However, in the great majority of patients, no such underlying cause can be identified. These cases have been classified as 'primary hypertension'. While the precise etiology of primary hypertension remains obscure, there is strong and convincing evidence that genetic factors together with environmental effects play a key role in its pathogenesis. Clinicians will continue to be limited to treatment approaches which are essentially palliative, rather than curative, until the pathogenesis of this disorder is much more clearly understood. Thus, efforts to understand the pathogenesis of primary hypertension have as their common goal the eventual development of specific therapeutic modalities aimed at curing or preventing this disease.

Physiological, endocrinological, pharmacological and neurobiological studies have identified a number of systems that affect vascular regulation and may, in certain forms of secondary hypertension, cause abnormal elevation of blood pressure. Historically, one of the first attempts to develop animal models for hypertension research was made by Tigerstedt and Bergman [1], who injected kidney extract (renin) into rabbits and observed a sustained increase of blood pressure. Subsequently, several models of experimental hypertension were developed by placing a lesion on vasculature, kidney, or other organs of otherwise healthy animals. The resulting hypertensinogenic dysfunction in many instances resembles specific hypertensive diseases in humans. Surgical manipulation of the kidney or of the renal artery, for example, results in renal hypertension.

Along similar lines, major advances in hypertension research have accompanied the development of genetically hypertensive rats [2]. Recently a single-gene defect has been successfully introduced into a hypertensive rat model [3]. Genetic modelling of animals is likely to expand in the future and will include recombinant DNA techniques.

Genetic hypertension in rats

The major difficulty in developing animal models for primary hypertension resides in the disease itself. Human primary hypertension may be considered a single entity from a clinical point of view. With respect to pathophysiology, natural history, response to treatment, and complications, however, it is a heterogeneous disease, and no uniform abnormality apart from the elevated blood pressure has been defined. In its early stages, even the classifications 'normotensive' and 'hypertensive' pose major problems because blood pressure is a quantitative trait, and the dividing line between normal variations and disease is arbitrary.

Table 1. Hypertensive rat strains

Name and origin of strain	Abbreviation	Major disturbances
Spontaneously hypertensive rat (Kyoto)	SHR	Neurogenic and cellular ionic transport abnormalities
Stroke-prone SHR (Kyoto)	SHRSP	Increased sympathetic tone
New Zealand genetically hypertensive (Dunedin)	GH	Increased peripheral resistance, Ca^{2+} metabolism, prostaglandins
Sabra hypertensive (Jerusalem)	SBH	Genetic predisposition to sodium retention
Milan hypertensive (Milan)	MHS	Cell-membrane defect resulting in abnormal kidney function
Dahl salt-sensitive (Brookhaven)		Gene-controlling adrenal steroids, abnormal pressure natriuresis, defect in
Non-inbred	DS	baroreceptor reflex, increased
Inbred	SS/Jr	sympathetic tone
Spontaneously hypertensive (Münster)	SHM	Membrane defect resulting in generalized disturbance in sodium handling
Lyon hypertensive (Lyon)	LH	Genetically determined defect in central nervous system function
SHRSP with hypothalamic diabetes insipidus (Heidelberg)	SHRSP-di	Increased sympathetic tone, absence of vasopressin
Fawn-hooded (Utrecht)	FH	Abnormal kidney function
Hypertensive transgenic rats	HTG	To be established

Genetically hypertensive rats have been obtained by genetic selection [2–9]. Inbred hypertensive strains provide a homogeneous population of hypertensive animals. The onset of high blood pressure occurs early, and complications occur at a predictable age if the environment is controlled. This is not the case in human primary hypertension, where age of onset varies widely and other factors are uncontrolled; its course, therefore, is much less predictable with respect to severity and complications. Thus, the homogeneity of inbred hypertensive rats is advantageous for scientific investigations, but caution must be exercised in extrapolating research results to humans because of the etiological heterogeneity of human hypertension.

The obvious and undisputed similarity of the hypertensive disease process in patients and in rats is its spontaneous development without a known cause in genetically predisposed subjects. The pathophysiological heterogeneity in humans finds its counterpart in the different strains of spontaneously hypertensive rats. *A priori*, it is virtually certain that the various inbred strains of hypertensive rats have trapped (i.e., genetically fixed) different, but overlapping subsets of specific genetic abnormalities causing high blood pressure.

Thus, one expects differences as well as similarities between strains (Table 1). The individual patient presenting with primary hypertension may have single or combined defects in salt sensitivity, renal electrolyte handling, cellular cation exchange, mineralocorticoid sensitivity, cellular calcium regulation, vascular reactivity, sympathetic tone, or neurogenic factors. Each strain or genetically hypertensive rats displays unique pathophysiological features linked to the development of hypertension which then often resemble disorders found in subgroups of hypertensive patients. Thus, the cause of hypertension in an individual hypertensive patient may closely resemble the disturbances found in one or more of the rat strains.

These hypertensive animals afford opportunities for investigations of basic mechanisms of blood pressure regulation that cannot be done in humans. The foremost advantage of animal studies lies in the comparability and reproducibility of study groups to a much greater degree than is possible in clinical studies. Invasive procedures that cannot be performed in humans, such as intracerebral injections, denervation, and nephrectomy, are feasible using animal models. The number of test animals can be readily predetermined, and the data show less scatter on account of the homogeneity of groups and absence of compliance problems.

Some general statements can be made concerning the similarities between genetically hypertensive rats and primary hypertension in humans:

1. The genetic component in both conditions is recognized, and the inheritance of blood pressure levels is probably polygenic.
2. The course of hypertension is similar. Blood pressure in humans and in rats rises with age.
3. The major cardiovascular complications in primary hypertension are also seen in rats.
4. Salt and other environmental factors contribute to the development of certain forms of human primary hypertension. In several models of genetic hypertension, the development of high blood pressure and its complications are also aggravated by these factors.
5. The efficacy of most antihypertensive agents and their combinations can be tested reliably in hypertensive rats. Drug testing is actually one of the major uses of genetically hypertensive rats because of their easy availability. In humans and in rats, the complications of hypertension, that is, the incidence of stroke, cardiac hypertrophy, renal failure, and malignant hypertension are equally reduced. This is a point of great importance when considering genetically hypertensive rats as animal models for studying human primary hypertension.

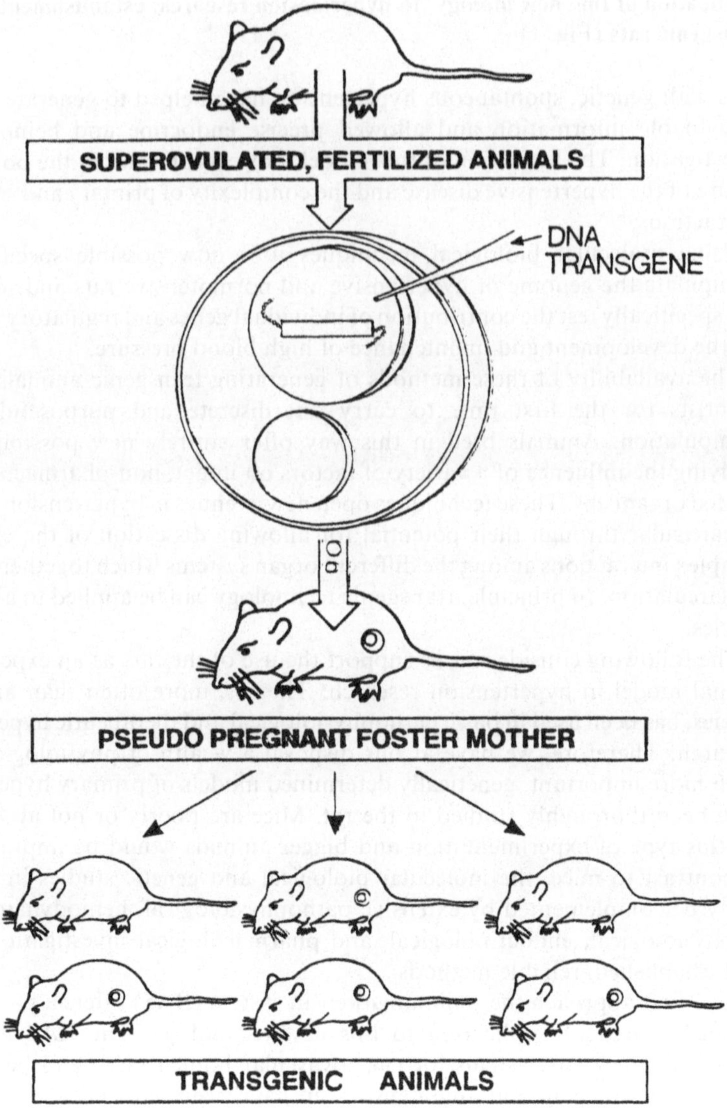

Fig. 1. Schematic outline of the production of transgenic animals. The most frequent technique for introducing genes into the germ line is direct microinjection of cloned DNA into pronuclei of fertilized eggs. These are obtained from superovulated females.

The DNA of the transgene is injected under the microscope into the pronucleus. The transfected egg is then implanted into a pseudopregnant foster mother. About 25% of the animals that are born carry one or more copies of the injected DNA. These animals are called transgenic and the foreign genes are referred to as transgenes. Because integration usually occurs prior to DNA replication, about 70% of the transgenic animals carry the transgenes in all their cells, including the germ cells. These animals can be used for further breeding of the new transgenic strain.

Application of the 'new biology' to hypertension research: establishment of transgenic rats (Fig. 1)

Rats with genetic, spontaneous hypertension have helped to generate a wealth of valuable information and allowed precise endocrine and hemodynamic investigation. The limitation of this model, however, resides in the polygenetic nature of the hypertensive disease and the complexity of primary and secondary interactions.

Using molecular biological techniques it is now possible specifically to manipulate the genome of hypertensive and normotensive rats and selectively and specifically test the contribution of individual genes and regulatory elements for the development and maintenance of high blood pressure.

The availability of these methods of generating transgenic animals enables scientists for the first time to carry out discrete and purposeful genetic manipulation. Animals bred in this way offer entirely new possibilities for studying the influence of a variety of factors on intact, non-pharmacologically treated organisms. These techniques open new avenues in hypertension research in particular through their potential for allowing dissection of the extremely complex interactions among the different organ systems which together regulate the circulation. In principle, transgenic technology can be applied to all animal species.

The following considerations support the use of the rats as an experimental animal model in hypertension research: The rat, more often than any other species, has been used in basic pathophysiological and therapeutic hypertension research. Therefore, we have at our disposal a wealth of physiological data. Even more important, genetically determined models of primary hypertension have been thoroughly studied in the rat. Mice are poorly or not at all suited for this type of experimentation and bigger animals would be impracticable. In contrast to mice, the molecular biological and genetic studies in rats can easily be complemented by extensive pathophysiological, hemodynamic, electrophysiological, endocrinological, and pharmacological investigations using well-established, reliable methods.

As a first approach the renin-angiotensin system (RAS) offers a particularly promising area of application to this new technology. The RAS is one of the most important systems for cardiovascular homeostasis; and besides the genes for both renin and angiotensinogen have been sequenced and are well characterized. Furthermore, the system has gained additional interest in the light of the newly recognized relationships between circulating and local tissue systems. Through transgenic modification of the RAS, important new insights about the pathogenesis of hypertension may be possible, which may result in major advances in the clinical management of hypertension.

This technique can be applied to virtually all blood pressure regulating systems, enzymes, peptides and receptors, as long as the respective genes are available. The establishment of transgenic rat models will combine the precision of this new biology with the versatility of the rat as an experimental animal for hypertension research. A most promising area of application is, for example, the transfection of rats with human genes allowing, for example, the development of specific inhibitors of human enzymes in transgenic rats. This would considerably facilitate drug development and reduce the ethical and financial problems involved in primate experimentation. Thus, transgenic animal techniques will provide research and industry with a new set of valuable and specific models for pathophysiological and therapeutic research.

Conclusions

Research oriented toward the clinical problem of hypertension has traditionally been limited by the inadequacy of *in vitro* or *in vivo* test systems which fail to provide a precise experimental counterpart for human disease. Meaningful generalizations from experimental models to human disease are difficult. Genetically hypertensive rats, however, display several important features found also in primary hypertension in humans, even if they provide only a narrow picture of the large spectrum of clinical hypertension. The overlap of similarities is broadened by the different kinds of hypertensive rat models available for research in this field today.

In the past, investigations using genetically hypertensive rats and other animal models have resulted in major advances in our understanding of the pathophysiology of hypertension. These valuable research resources will continue to aid in finding the source of human hypertension and ultimately preventing this disease. In the future, application of the 'new biology' to hypertension research using recombinant DNA technology and, in particular, the establishment of transgenic rats, will provide powerful and specific new animal models for hypertension research.

The obvious advantages of this type of animal research make mandatory a concentrated effort to apply and further develop its use as a tool for hypertension research. It is only through basic research and the responsible use of all available *in vitro* and *in vivo* methods, that new and better treatment modalitites for hypertension will be designed. Ultimately, we may even be able to prevent this disease altogether and thus eliminate a major cause of cardiovascular morbidity and mortality.

References

1. Tigerstedt R, Bergman PG (1898) Niere und Kreislauf. *Scand Arch Physiol* 8: 223–279
2. Rascher W, Clough D, Ganten D (Eds) *Hypertensive mechanisms: the spontaneously hypertensive rat as a model to study human hypertension.* Stuttgart: Schauttauer Verlag, 1982, pp 777–802
3. Ganten U, Rascher W, Lang RE, *et al.* (1983) Development of a new strain of spontaneously hypertensive rats homozygous for hypothalamic diabetes insipidus. *Hypertension* 5 (suppl I): I-119–I-128

4. Yamori K, Okamoto K (1970) Zymogram analyses of various organs from spontaneously hypertensive rats. *Lab Invest* 22: 206–211
5. Rapp JP, Dahl LK (1972) Mendelian inheritance of 18- and 11β-steroid hydroxylase activities in the adrenals of rats genetically susceptible or resistant to hypertension. *Endocrinology* 90: 1435–1446
6. Tanase H (1979) Genetic control of blood pressure in spontaneously hypertensive rats (SHR). *Exp Animals* 28: 519–530
7. Rapp JP (1982) A genetic locus (Hyp-2) controlling vascular smooth muscle response in spontaneously hypertensive rats. *Hypertension* 4: 459–467
8. Okamoto K, Yamori Y, Ooshima A, Park C, Haebara H, Matsumoto M. Establishment of the inbred strain of the spontaneously hypertensive rat and genetic factors involved in hypertension. In: Okamoto K (Ed) *Spontaneous hypertension: its pathogenesis and complications.* Tokyo: Igaku Shoin 1972: 1–8
9. Udenfriend S, Bumpus FM, Foster HL, *et al.* (1976) Spontaneously hypertensive rats: guidelines for breeding, care and use. *ILAR News* 19(3): G1–G20

Animal experiments and recent progress in thrombosis research

GIOVANNI DE GAETANO, CHIARA CERLETTI, ANDREINA POGGI and MARIA BENEDETTA DONATI

Research Institute for Pharmacology 'Mario Negri', Southern Section of the Santa Maria Imbaro, Italy

Thrombosis and vascular disease

Thrombosis is a complex, multifactorial process characterized by partial or total occlusion of a vessel. In the arterial vascular tree, thrombosis is closely related to atherosclerosis, another complex process, characterized by the formation of an atheromatous plaque on the vascular wall.

It is presently accepted that vascular damage is the first event in both thrombosis and atherosclerosis. Circulating blood platelets rapidly adhere to injured vessel wall and release intracellular constituents such as adenosine diphosphate and thromboxane A2, which induce passing platelets to aggregate on the top of adhering cells. Plasma membranes of activated platelets offer a catalytic surface to blood coagulation factors which lead to rapid generation of fibrin: this is the insoluble end product of blood clotting and constitutes the major structure of thrombi. Fibrin generation induces local activation of the fibrinolytic system, which may eventually lead to clot dissolution.

White and red blood cells and plasma lipid constituents such as cholesterol also contribute to thrombosis and atherosclerosis, as well as to the hemodynamic and rheological characteristics of the circulation in any given vessel [1, 2].

In view of the pathogenetic mechanism of thrombosis involving different cellular, plasmatic and vascular components, it is not surprising that many therapeutic approaches have been developed in the attempt to prevent and/or reduce its clinical consequences. Thrombosis constitutes the major pathological finding of severe ischemic arterial disease, such as acute myocardial infarction, stroke and occlusive disease of the lower limbs.

Recently controlled clinical trials involving about 100,000 patients with different thrombotic diseases have shown that drugs inhibiting platelet function (e.g. aspirin), or blood coagulation (e.g. heparin) or activating fibrinolysis (e.g. streptokinase) may significant reduce both non fatal and fatal complications of ischemic vascular diseases [3–7].

Despite these encouraging therapeutic results, many problems remain in the physiopathology, biochemistry, pharmacology, diagnosis, treatment and

S. Garattini (ed.), The Importance of Animal Experimentation for Safety and Biomedical Research, 97–109.

epidemiology of thrombosis: the triggers and the mechanisms of vascular injury *in vivo* are still largely obscure, as is the role of possible interactions between platelets and polymorphonuclear leukocytes in the damaged area in ischemic tissues. Besides, the mechanism of action of the few available antithrombotic drugs is not yet completely elucidated [1, 2].

Thus a tremendous research effort is required to obtain a significant modification of the natural history of thrombotic disease in future years. Besides other considerations, the socio-economic impact of thrombotic disease should also be taken into account as myocardial infarction affects mainly middle aged active men, often at the top of their productive activity, and cerebral stroke is frequently followed by severely disabling consequences.

As an example, every year in Italy about 100,000 people have an acute myocardial infarction; 30,000 patients die within the first few seconds or minutes, before reaching a hospital. About 9,000 patients die during the first 3–5 weeks in hospital, while an other 6,000 die within one year from the first symptoms. A drug preventing overall mortality after myocardial infarction by *only* 20% would spare at least 9,000 lives each year.

From these brief introductory remarks, it appears that a better understanding of the thrombotic process and substantial improvement in its prevention and therapy will only result from a multidisciplinary approach involving different methods and models and complementary skills.

In the framework of the present discussion on the use of animals in biomedical research, we shall present a few examples mainly deriving from our personal research experience in the field of thrombosis and antithrombotic drugs. In particular we shall discuss the following topics:

1. How animal experiments were essential in the development of new concepts, from the role of vascular cells in thrombogenesis to the importance of platelets in atherogenesis;
2. How new developments in the clinical use of 'old' drugs such as aspirin and heparin in thrombosis prevention benefited from animal-derived information;
3. How future developments in the field of thrombosis can already be anticipated by the use of monoclonal antibodies against platelet membrane glycoproteins, for instance, or the identification of RGD-containing peptide sequences;
4. How the discovery of a cysteine-protease with procoagulant activity first identified in rabbit and murine models of cancer might lead to novel approaches to the treatment of patients with cancer or blood clotting disorders;
5. Finally, how the definition and usefulness of an animal 'model' is not necessarily limited by species-related peculiarities.

Animal experiments and new concepts in thrombosis research

In the last ten years several new ideas and innovative hypotheses have been developed in this field. A very important cultural revolution resides in the concept that blood vessels are not 'inert containers' (such as the unwettable plastic bags used for blood transfusion), but a well equipped 'biochemical laboratory' able to synthesize and/or release a number of active constituents in response to adequate stimuli. Some of these constituents regulate the tone of the vessel itself, others interact with blood platelets, blood coagulation or the fibrinolytic system.

The discovery of prostacyclin... The discovery in 1976 of prostacyclin (identified as a prostaglandin of the 2-series, namely PGI_2) was the result of a bioassay based on a cascade of animal tissues in a pharmacological bath [8]. PGI_2 is a powerful vasodilator and platelet aggregation inhibitor. Shortly thereafter the same investigators who had found PGI_2 in animal vessels reported that human vessels too were able to synthesize and release a substance identical to PGI_2 [9]. Our group was soon interested by this discovery and obtained in rats (fed a hypercholesterolemic diet) the first data suggesting a link between vascular PGI_2 and atherosclerosis [10]. This link was confirmed in human atheromatous plaques found to be defective in PGI_2 generating capacity [11].

... and the pathogenesis of uremic bleeding. At about the same time we had started an ambitious project aimed at understanding the complex hemorrhagic complications associated with the uremic condition [12]. It was obvious to measure PGI_2 generation in vessels obtained during the application of an artero-venous shunt to patients with renal failure undergoing hemodialysis. These patients suffered frequent bleeding complications and the elevated PGI_2 levels found in their vessels offered a new, unexpected clue to an original interpretation of the complex hemostatic derangement associated with uremia [13]. In subsequent years an Austrian group reported that rats with experimentally induced uremia also had increased production of vascular PGI_2 [14]. These animals, similarly to uremic patients, have a prolonged bleeding time and this is the most reliable clinical test at present available to evaluate the hemorrhagic tendency in an individual.

It has now been reported that conjugated estrogens correct the abnormal bleeding times both in patients and in rats with uremia [15, 16]. Current studies aimed at elucidating the mechanism of action of these compounds will include the use of the model of the uremic rat.

... and the treatment of patients with hemolytic uremic syndrome. We were at the same time interested by a special form of uremia accompanied by severe hemolysis and characterized by diffuse thrombosis of the microcirculation. This is called hemolytic uremic syndrome (HUS) and is very similar if not identical to another clinical condition referred to as thrombotic thrombocytopenic purpura (TTP). In vascular specimens from patients with either HUS or TTP, we found a consistent, severe deficiency of PGI_2 generation [17].

During the same period, the interesting observation was made by British investigators that porcine vascular cells in culture were able to produce PGI_2 and that such a production could be markedly increased by incubation with normal human plasma. Following this experimental observation [18], we found that plasma from patients with HUS/TTP, unlike plasma from healthy subjects failed to stimulate rat vascular PGI_2 production *in vitro* [19]. Infusion of normal plasma in one of these patients resulted in a dramatic improvement of both laboratory data and clinical symptoms and in restoration of plasma PGI_2 capacity. Many other patients with HUS/TTP have since been successfully treated with plasma infusion. This approach is still considered today the most effective therapy for such complex, often fatal syndromes [20].

In conclusion, the discovery of PGI_2 in an experimental system based on animal tissues became the conceptual and experimental trigger to obtain results useful for the understanding and the management of two serious clinical conditions associated with renal insufficiency. The hypothesis that patients with HUS/TTP could be treated with plasma infusion to restore impaired vascular PGI_2 production would hardly have been put forward without animal experimentation. It cannot be excluded that plasma infusion will be found to be effective by a mechanism unrelated to PGI_2 synthesis and it will certainly be replaced by more specific and effective treatments. Nevertheless, the contribution of the PGI_2-hypothesis to the solution of a mysterious chapter in medical history should not be underestimated.

From Nerve Growth Factor (NGF) to the role of blood platelets and vascular cells in atherosclerosis. According to modern concepts, blood platelets play an essential role in the pathogenesis of atherosclerosis, particularly in the formation of advanced lesions. Platelets do not adhere to intact endothelial cells under physiological conditions; however, when they accumulate at the site of vascular injury, they undergo a secretion reaction which contributes to progression of the atherosclerotic lesion in a number of ways. The most significant appears to be secretion of a platelet-derived growth factor (PDGF) [21]. Human PDGF is an approximately 30,000 mol. weight protein composed of two polypeptide chains linked by disulfide bonds. The existence of PDGF was suggested in 1974 when it was shown that human serum derived from platelet-rich blood but not that obtained from platelet-poor blood, stimulated the proliferation of primate (monkeys) arterial smooth muscle cells in culture [22].

It was subsequently discovered that the active mitogenic material present in serum was PDGF. However, the concept that cells may secrete molecules acting upon the growth of other cells was first generated in the Fifties by the finding that some mouse tumors enhanced growth of chick embryo ganglia and that this effect was due to a humoral factor released in the circulation of the host by these grafted tumors. In view of its powerful nerve growth promoting activity this factor was named NGF by Rita Levi-Montalcini [23]. More recently, an endothelial cell derived growth factor (ECDGF) has been shown in the culture medium of arterial endothelial cells from many different animal species [24]. The importance of ECDGF in the pathogenesis of atherosclerosis remains to be established. The picture is complicated by the observation that cultured endothelial cells also secrete a substance similar to heparin, which inhibits the growth of vascular smooth muscle cells [25]. The family of PDGF has been enriched in the last few years by the discovery and identification of other proteins such as TGFβ [26] and EGF. The latter was first noticed in 1960 in snake venoms and in mouse submaxillary glands and subsequently isolated from human urine in 1975 [27].

Animal experiments and new developments in the search for antithrombotic drugs

The discovery of PGI_2 mentioned in the previous section was rapidly followed by the observation that when given intravenously to normal rats aspirin inhibited its generation [28]. Our finding, together with similar data from other laboratories, constituted the experimental basis for the so-called 'aspirin dilemma' [29].

A chapter in the 90-year 'aspirin story': the 'aspirin dilemma'. PGI_2 is generated from a precursor fatty acid, arachidonic acid, through the formation of unstable cyclic endoperoxides, by the enzyme cyclo-oxygenase. The same biochemical pathway gives origin in platelets to thromboxane A2 (TxA2), another prostanoid with proaggregatory and vaso-constrictory properties. As expected, synthesis of TxA2 was inhibited by aspirin. As platelet aggregation and vasoconstriction were considered two important mechanisms in the pathogenesis of vascular occlusion, it was feared that the potential antithrombotic effect of aspirin, possibly associated with platelet TxA2 suppression by this drug could be counteracted by concomitant PGI_2 inhibition in vascular cells.

In vitro experiments comparing human cultured endothelial cells and blood platelets indicated substantially similar susceptibility to aspirin inhibition [30], a conclusion in good agreement with *in vivo* data obtained after *intravenous* administration of aspirin to normal rats [31]. Platelet TxA2 and abdominal aorta PGI_2 synthesis was comparably prevented by aspirin. However, when aspirin was given *orally*, a marked dissociation was found between the inhibition of platelet TxA2 and vascular PGI_2. The latter was spared by doses of aspirin completely suppressing the former. It was therefore suggested that the rapid hydrolysis of oral aspirin during absorption and the first passage through the liver would result in presystemic acetylation of circulating blood platelets within the gastrointestinal microvasculature; in contrast, peripheral vessels would preferentially come in contact with salicylate, the inactive hydrolysis product of aspirin. This hypothesis was verified in rats by showing that:

a) PGI_2 generation by the portal vein, a presystemic vessel, but not by the vena cava, a systemic vessel, was prevented by oral aspirin as effectively as blood platelet arachidonate metabolism [31];

b) Institution of an experimental porta-cava shunt resulted in a substantial reduction of the presystemic effect of oral aspirin on platelet TxA2 generation [32].

More recently, a meta-analysis of 19 clinical trials with aspirin in the secondary prevention of vascular events found no significant difference between doses of aspirin which, based on *in vitro* data, should have affected vascular PGI_2 generation differently [3]. Measurements of urinary excretion of PGI_2 metabolites in patients with cerebrovascular disorder, given either 300 of 1200 mg daily of oral aspirin, failed to demonstrate any significant inhibition of that peripheral parameter (C. Cerletti *et al.*, unpublished). Possibly, even chronic treatment with high dose aspirin does not result in a clinically relevant 'aspirin dilemma'.

In conclusion this brief 'aspirin story' clearly shows that *in vitro* data may give information not consistent with the *in vivo* events in an intact individual. The possibility of measuring PGI_2 generation directly on vascular specimens from different districts in the rat was of primary importance for a more rational use of aspirin in humans.

Heparin: animal experiments and the re-discovery of an old anticoagulant drug. The antithrombotic activity and the hemorrhagic potential of heparin have been generally attributed to its well-known anticoagulant activity. Little emphasis has so far been laid on the possible interference of heparin with primary hemostasis. Some years ago the hypothesis that heparin affects primary hemostasis by inhibiting platelet function was based on (somewhat neglected) observations that heparin prolongs bleeding time in human healthy volunteers [33]. Pangrazzi *et al.* [34] studying the effects of heparin in rats, suggested that mechanisms other than those involved in coagulation might be affected by some low molecular weight heparin components, which are not removed during the fractionation of high molecular weight heparin. One of these components was subsequently identified by nuclear magnetic resonance as EDTA, a calcium chelating agent [35]. As a consequence, the preparation of some heparins for clinical use has been modified to ensure removal of this dangerous contaminant.

More recently, Borowska *et al.* [36] found a close association between the degree of hemorrhagic potential of four low molecular weight fractions – evaluated *in vivo* with an experimental model of bleeding – and the extent of inhibition of platelet aggregation *in vitro* and *ex vivo* with the same materials. The mechanism of action of low molecular weight heparins in inhibiting platelet aggregations remains to be elucidated. Since low molecular weight heparin preparations prolonged bleeding time in animals pretreated with high doses of aspirin (which fully blocked platelet and vascular cyclo-oxygenase activity), it seems unlikely that this compound acts by modulating the thromboxane–prostacyclin balance. Interestingly enough, those low molecular weight heparin fractions prolonging bleeding time were also able to prevent platelet aggregation induced by combined stimuli, an experimental system in which aspirin is reportedly ineffective.

Whatever its mechanism of action, heparin and some low molecular weight preparations may affect platelet function. A novel approach to platelet inhibition may thus be generated by research on heparin, the most famous anticoagulant drug over the last fifty years.

Animal experiments and future developments in thrombosis research

One of the biggest research impacts in recent years has been the identification of surface glycoproteins that mediate platelet adhesion and aggregation [37]. The better understanding of the molecular basis for platelet function has already generated some new ideas on the possible modulation of the role of platelets in thrombosis. This includes the use of monoclonal antibodies against platelet glycoproteins such as the GPIIb/IIIa complex and competitive inhibition between adhesive proteins and RGD-containing peptides. Adhesive proteins include fibrinogen, von Willebrand factor, fibronectin and other proteins consisting of common or very similar subunits [38].

Monoclonal antibodies against platelet membrane glycoproteins. Intravenous administration in animals of monoclonal antibodies against the GPIIb/IIIa complex – the glycoproteins mainly responsible for fibrinogen binding to platelet surface – resulted in time- and dose-dependent prolongation of bleeding time, inhibition of platelet aggregation induced by ADP or collagen and reduction of platelet deposition onto acutely placed Dacron vascular grafts [39]. Interestingly enough, bleeding times were prolonged acutely and remained abnormal for at least 24–48 hours. Injection of an anti-platelet GpIIb/IIIa monoclonal antibody to dogs accelerated lysis induced by recombinant tissue-type plasminogen activator (rt-PA) and prevented reocclusion in experimental coronary artery thrombosis. However, the same antibody failed to potentiate thrombolysis with rt-PA of venous thrombi [40], suggesting it acts specifically against platelet-mediated arterial thrombosis.

RGD-containing peptide sequences. The ability of platelets to bind fibrinogen and related adhesion proteins, such as fibronectin, appears to depend on a short, hydrophilic amino-acid sequence (Arg-Gly-Asp, RGD) located in the cell binding domain of the fibrinogen molecule [37, 38]. Synthetic peptides containing this sequence may act as competitive reversible inhibitors of the interaction between fibrinogen and platelets. They have been used in several laboratories to study adhesive interactions involved not only in platelet function, but also in experimental metastasis. Such peptides prevented the binding of fibrinogen, fibronectin and von Willebrand factor to activated human platelets and prevented platelet aggregation by ADP or thrombin. They also prevented the formation of lung colonies in mice injected with murine melanoma cells [41]. Studies in progress (A. Poggi *et al.* unpublished) indicate that there are important species differences in the ability of the RGD-peptides to block platelet fibrinogen receptors. While human and mouse platelet aggregation was prevented by some RGD peptides, rat platelet aggregation was not. Our results confirm and extend recent findings that rabbit or rat platelet reactions were not influenced by RGD-peptides, while human platelet reactions were markedly reduced [42].

These findings should caution against general application of the concept of RGD as a common cell attachment sequence. Another note of caution is related to the fact that the RGD sequency may not be the sole recognition site within each of the adhesive proteins. On the other hand, in view of the broad range of adhesive reactions mediated by proteins containing the RGD sequence, future approaches to platelet inhibition might be limited by unwanted reactions at the level of other cells. Moreover, the presently available peptides have a very short half-life and must be administered intravenously. Neither property is compatible with a drug to be given for years to large populations.

As the GPIIb/IIIa receptor on the platelet surface is only exposed after cell activation, monoclonal antibodies and/or RGD-peptides might be used as selective carriers of antiplatelet drugs. In this way aspirin might be able to selectively acetylate activated platelets, while sparing the function of other platelets which might secure normal hemostasis. Aspirin carried to platelet receptors would reduce ischemic disease without increasing hemorrhagic risk, as occurred, in contrast, in primary prevention trials recently reported (see ref. [4]).

Animal experiments and the cancer procoagulant

Cancer procoagulant is a newly identified activator of the blood clotting system, found in a number of human malignancies, as a consequence of more than ten years of research work in murine tumor metastasis models.

The search for a peculiar procoagulant expressed by some tumor cells started from the observation that oral anticoagulants such as warfarin, but not other anticoagulants such as heparin, were able to prevent lung metastasis growth from solid tumors implanted in different murine systems [43, 44]. Evidence was obtained of the involvement of vitamin K in this effect since experimental metastasis was also prevented by a vitamin K-deficient diet and reverted to control levels on addition of vitamin K to the diet [44, 45]. On the basis of these studies, the hypothesis was put forward that an hitherto unknown vitamin K-dependent activity might be closely associated with human tumor cells; this activity was able to promote fibrin deposition in the tumor microenvironment by activating blood clotting through a peculiar mechanism, i.e. direct activation of coagulation factor X. It was a cysteine protease, not a serine protease like most of the known clotting factors, and needed calcium ions for its biological activity, like all known vitamin K-dependent proteins. But the most interesting characteristic of cancer procoagulant was that in all experimental models tested its presence and/or degree of activity was closely associated with the metastatic potential of the cells [46]. This observation offers on the one hand a clue to the antimetastatic effect of warfarin and congeners, which is at present being investigated in clinical trials; on the other hand, cancer procoagulant has now been identified in human malignancies (melanoma, breast cancer, acute promyelocytic leukemia) and found to be selectively associated with the malignant phenotype [47, 48].

Only one non-neoplastic tissue has been found to express a protein similar to cancer procoagulant, human amniochorial tissue [49], stressing the concept that this protease is only detectable in undifferentiated or de-differentiated cells.

Research is presently going on to verify whether cancer procoagulant can be regarded as a new marker of malignancy, in the serum of tumor patients and in the bone marrow of acute leukemia patients.

Cancer procoagulant has a peculiar mode of action in the clotting cascade; availability of the purified protein and the knowledge of its primary structure will open new possibilities in the diagnosis and treatment of some clotting disorders. Indeed, it is conceivable that the production of cancer procoagulant by recombinant technology could provide a new 'hemostatic' tool for the treatment of hemorrhagic disorders; the protein could also be useful as a reagent for the diagnosis of factor X abnormalities.

Animal models and human models in thrombosis research

People not involved in thrombosis research may well believe that:

a) animals are too different from man to give reliable information on human thrombotic disease or its treatment
b) even if some mechanisms are similar in animals and man, the usefulness of the animal model is anyway reduced by the fact that 'man is not a 70 kg rat'.

A few examples will show that species differences are often more useful than similarities, but also that important biological differences through the human species itself, providing interesting human models. It is known for example, that the rat is fairly resistant to atherosclerosis induced by a cholesterol-rich diet while the rabbit develops atherosclerotic lesions in the same experimental conditions [10]. The mechanisms by which rats are protected against atheromatous plaque formation are probably more interesting than those involved in mimicking the human vascular lesion. It is of interest to note that human [9] and rabbit [50] veins produce larger amounts of prostacyclin than the respective arteries, while rat [28] vessels behave in the opposite way. As already mentioned, prostacyclin is a natural powerful antiplatelet and vasodilatory compound [8]. Whether vascular prostacyclin generation is a mechanism protecting individuals against atherosclerosis remains to be established, but this hypothesis has already stimulated intensive experimental and clinical research.

As far as acute myocardial infarction is concerned there is still no satisfactory explanation of its different incidence between males and females (4:1). The recent GISSI trial [6] has shown that in hospital mortality of female patients with myocardial infarction is markedly higher than that of comparable males; thrombolytic treatment with streptokinase however was significantly effective in both males and females.

Although female sexual hormones play a defensive role against coronary artery disease, groups of females with and without this disease should be carefully investigated as useful 'models' for myocardial infarction in men.

A third example is given by the epidemiological observation that clinical manifestations of atherosclerotic vascular disease are rarer among Greenland Eskimos than among Eskimos living in Denmark [51].

It has been proposed that Eskimos benefit from eating more fish, thus having a high intake of poly-unsaturated fatty acids of the omega-3 family, mainly eicosapentaenoic acid (EPA). When normal Western diets are supplemented with fish or fish oil, EPA takes the place of arachidonic acid in the phospholipids of platelet membranes. This is associated with decreasing platelet aggregation and prolongation of bleeding time. Knapp *et al.* [52] have investigated how endogenous prostanoid metabolism was influenced by dietary supplementation with EPA. After four weeks of fish oil supplementation a slight but significant prolongation of bleeding time was observed both in healthy volunteers and in patients with atherosclerosis. Urinary excretion of prostanoid metabolites of the 2-series was markedly reduced in patients, while only urinary TxB_2 but not PGI_2 metabolite excretion was decreased in healthy volunteers. The 'biochemical selectivity' of fish oil in reducing thromboxane synthesis, while sparing prostacyclin synthesis, is of interest but cannot be easily explained. Perhaps dietary EPA supplementation might be associated with aspirin to increase the 'biochemical selectivity' of this drug, which is related to its peculiar pharmacokinetics. One additional potentially antithrombotic effect of poly-unsaturated fatty acids is linked to their capacity to lower total serum cholesterol and triglycerides [53]. Although several questions have to be answered before fish-oil dietary supplementation can be proposed on a large scale to Western populations, the potential benefit of this dietary approach to prevent thrombosis and atherosclerosis is of the greatest interest.

Conclusions

In conclusion, animal experiments should not be regarded as simplistic tools to extrapolate experimental findings to clinical conditions or to screen antithrombotic compounds that way effective in man. The use of animals in thrombosis research is an essential part of a multistep strategy to develop innovative concepts, new methods and possibly new surgical and medical therapeutic approaches.

Acknowledgements

The Authors acknowledge the financial support of the Italian National Research Council (CNR, Convenzione con il Consorzio Mario Negri Sud). Judy Baggott, Silvia Falcone and Daniela Spadano helped prepare the manuscript.

References

1. de Gaetano G, Cerletti C, Dejana E, Vermylen J (1986) Current issues in thrombosis prevention with antiplatelet drugs. *Drugs* 31: 517–549
2. de Gaetano G, Bertelè V, Cerletti C (1987) Pharmacology of antiplatelet drugs. In: MacIntyre D.E. and Gordon J.L. (Eds) *Platelets in biology and pathology* III, Elsevier, Amsterdam pp 515–573
3. Antiplatelet Trialists' Collaboration (1988) Secondary prevention of vascular disease by prolonged antiplatelet treatment. *Br Med J* 296: 320–331
4. de Gaetano G (1988) Primary prevention of vascular disease by aspirin. *Lancet* 1: 1093–1094
5. Collins R, Scrimgeour A, Yusuf S, Peto R (1988) Reductjon in fatal pulmonary embolism and venous thrombosis by perioperative administration of subcutaneous heparin: Overview of results of randomized trials in general, orthopedic, and urology surgery. *N Engl J Med* 318: 1162–1173
6. GISSI (Gruppo Italiano per lo Studio della Streptochinasi nell'Infarto miocardico) (1986) Effectiveness of intravenous thrombolytic treatment in acute myocardial infarction. *Lancet* I: 379
7. ISIS-2 Collaborative Group (1988) Randomised trial of intravenous streptokinase, oral aspirin, both or neither among 17,189 cases of suspected acute myocardial infarction. *Lancet* II: 349–360
8. Moncada S, Gryglewski R, Bunting S, Vane JR (1976) An enzyme isolated from arteries transforms prostaglandin endoperoxides to an unstable substance that inhibits platelet aggregation. *Nature* 263: 663–665
9. Moncada S, Higgs EA, Vane JR (1977) Human arterial and venous tissues generate prostacyclin (prostaglandin X), a potent inhibitor of platelet aggregation. *Lancet* I: 18–20
10. Villa S, Mysliwiec M, de Gaetano G (1977) Prostacyclin and atherosclerosis in rats. *Lancet* II: 1216–1217
11. D'Angelo V, Villa S, Mysliwiec M, Donati MB, de Gaetano G (1978) Defective fibrinolytic and prostacyclin-like activity in human atheromatous plaques. *Thromb Haemost* 39: 535–536
12. Remuzzi G, Livio M, Marchiaro G, Mecca G, de Gaetano G (1978) Bleeding in renal failure: Altered platelet function in chronic uraemia only partially corrected by haemodialysis. *Nephron* 22: 347–353
13. Remuzzi G, Cavenaghi AE, Mecca G, Donati MB, de Gaetano G (1977) Prostacyclin-like activity and bleeding in renal failure. Lancet II: 1195–1197.
14. Leithner CH, Winter M, Silbauer K, Wagner O, Pinggera W, Sinzinger H (1978) Enhanced prostacyclin availability of blood vessels in uraemic humans and rats. In: Robinson RHB, Hawkins JB (Eds) *Dialysis transplantation nephrology*. Proceedings of the 15th Congress of European Dialysis and Transplant Association. Tunbridge Wells: *Pitman Medical*, 418–422
15. Remuzzi G (1988) Bleeding in renal failure. *Lancet* I: 1205–1208
16. Zoja C, Viganò G, Bergamelli A, Benigni A (1989) Prolonged bleeding time and increased vascular prostacyclin in rats with chronic renal failure: effects of conjugated estrogens. *J Lab Clin Med*, in press.
17. Remuzzi G, Livio M, Cavenaghi AE, Marchesi D, Mecca G, Donati MB, de Gaetano G

(1978) Unbalanced prostaglandin synthesis and plasma factors in uraemic bleeding. A hypothesis. *Thromb Res* 13: 531–536.
18. MacIntyre DE, Pearson JD, Gordon JL (1978) Localisation and stimulation of prostacyclin production in vascular cells. *Nature* 271: 549.
19. Donati MB, Misiani R, Marchesi D, Livio M, Mecca G, Remuzzi G, de Gaetano G (1980) Hemolytic-uremic syndrome, prostaglandins, and plasma factors. In: Remuzzi G, Mecca G, and de Gaetano G (Eds) *Hemostasis, Prostaglandins and Renal Disease*, Raven Press, New York: 283–290.
20. Remuzzi G (1987) Thrombotic thrombocytopenic purpura and allied disorders. In: Verstraete M, Vermylen J, Lijnen R and Arnout J (Eds) *Thrombosis and Haemostasis*, Leuven University Press, Leuven: 673–708
21. Ross R (1986) The pathogenesis of atherosclerosis - an update. *N Engl J Med* 314: 488–500
22. Ross R, Glomset J, Kariya B, Harker L (1974) A platelet-dependent serum factor that stimulates the proliferation of arterial smooth muscle cells in vitro. *Proc Natl Acad Sci* USA 71: 1207–1210
23. Calissano P, Cattaneo A, Biocca S, Aloe L, Mercanti D, Levi-Montalcini R (1984) The nerve growth factor. Established findings and controversial aspects. *Exp Cell Res* 154: 1–9
24. Gajdusek CM, Di Corleto PE, Ross R, Schwartz SM (1980) An endothelial cell-derived growth factor. *J Cell Biol* 85: 476–472
25. Castellot JJ Jr, Addonizio ML, Rosenberg R, Karnowsky MJ (1981) Cultured endothelial cells produce a heparinlike inhibitor of smooth muscle cell growth. *J Cell Biol* 90: 372–379
26. Sporn MB, Roberts AB, Wakefield M, Assoian RK (1986) Transforming growth factor β: biological function and chemical structure. *Science* 233: 532–534
27. Carpenter G, Zendegui JZ (1986) Epidermal growth factor, its receptors, and related proteins. *Exp Cell Res* 164: 1–10
28. Villa S, de Gaetano G (1977) Prostacyclin-like activity in rat vascular tissues. Fast, long-lasting inhibition by treatment with lysine acetylsalicylate. *Prostaglandins* 14: 1117–1124.
29. de Gaetano G, Cerletti C, Bertelè V (1982) Pharmacology of antiplatelet drugs and clinical trials on thrombosis prevention: a difficult link. *Lancet* II: 974–977
30. Bertelè V, Falanga A, Tomasiak M, Dejana E, Cerletti C, de Gaetano G (1983) Platelet thromboxane synthetase inhibitors with low doses of aspirin: Possible resolution of the 'aspirin dilemma'. *Science* 220: 517–519
31. Cerletti C, Gambino MC, Garattini S, de Gaetano G (1986) Biochemical selectivity of oral versus intravenous aspirin in rats. Inhibition by oral aspirin of cyclooxygenase activity in platelets and presystemic but not systemic vessels. *J Clin Invest* 78: 323–326
32. Gambino MC, Passaghe S, Chen ZM, Bucchi F, Gori G, Latini R, de Gaetano G, Cerletti C (1988) Selectivity of oral aspirin as an inhibitor of platelet vs. vascular cyclooxygenase activity is reduced by portacaval shunt in rats. *J Pharmacol Exp Ther* 245: 287–290
33. Heiden D, Mielke CH Jr, Rodvien R (1977) Impairment by heparin of primary haemostasis and platelet (^{14}C)-hydroxytryptamine release. *Br J Haematol* 36: 427–436
34. Pangrazzi J, Abbadini M, Zametta M, Naggi A, Torri G, Casu B, Donati MB (1985) Antithrombotic and bleeding effects of low molecular weight heparin fraction. *Biochem Pharmacol* 34: 3305–3308
35. Casu B, Naggi A, Oreste P, Torri G, Pangrazzi J, Maggi A, Abbadini M, Donati MB (1987) Bleeding effects associated with heparin contaminants. *Lancet* I: 1088
36. Borowska A, Lauri D, Maggi A, Dejana E, de Gaetano G, Donati MB, Pangrazzi J (1987) Impairment of primary haemostasis by low molecular weight heparins in rats. *Br J Haematol* 68: 339–344
37. Nurden AT (1987) Platelet membrane glycoproteins and their clinical aspects. In: Verstraete M, Vermylen J, Lijnen R and Arnout J (Eds) *Thrombosis and Haemostasis*. Leuven University Press, Leuven: 93–125
38. Phillips DR, Charo IF, Parise LV, Fitzgerald L (1988) The platelet membrane glycoprotein

IIb-IIIa complex. *Blood* 71: 831–843

39. Hanson SR, Pareti FI, Ruggeri ZM, Marzec UM, Kunicki TJ, Montgomery RR, Zimmermann TS, Harker L (1988) Effects of monoclonal antibodies against the platelet glycoprotein IIb/IIa complex on thrombosis and hemostasis in the baboon. *J Clin Invest* 8: 149–158.
40. Gold HK, Coller BS, Yasuda T, Saito T, Fallon JT, Guerrero L, Leinbach RC, Ziskind AA, Collen D (1988) Rapid and sustained coronary artery recanalization with combined bolus injection of recombinant tissue-type plasminogen activator and monoclonal antiplatelet GPIIb/IIIa antibody in a canine preparation. *Circulation* 77: 670–677
41. Humphries MJ, Olden K, Yamada KM (1986) A synthetic peptide from fibronectin inhibits experimental metastasis of murine melanoma cells. *Science* 233: 467–470
42. Harfenist EJ, Packham MA, Mustard JF (1988) Effects of the cell adhesion peptide, Arg-Gly-Asp-Ser, on responses of washed platelets from humans, rabbits, and rats. *Blood* 71: 132–136
43. Poggi A, Mussoni L, Kornblihtt L, Ballabio E, de Gaetano G, Donati MB (1978) Warfarin enantiomers anticoagulation, and experimental tumor metastasis. *Lancet* I: 163–164
44. Colucci M, Delaini F, De Bellis Vitti G, Locati D, Poggi A, Semeraro N, Donati MB (1983) Warfarin inhibits both procoagulant activity and metastatic capacity of Lewis Lung Carcinoma cells: role of vitamin K deficiency. *Biochem Pharmacol* 32: 1689–1691
45. Donati MB, Roncaglioni MC, Falanga A, Casali B, Semeraro N (1986) Vitamin K-dependent procoagulant in cancer cells: a potential target for the antimetastatic effect of warfarin? *Haemostasis* 16: 288–294
46. Falanga A, Bolognese AP, Casali B, Roncaglioni MC, Donati MB (1987) Several murine metastatising tumours possess a cysteine proteinase with cancer procoagulant characteristics. *Int J Cancer* 39: 774–777
47. Donati MB, Gambacorti-Passerini C, Casali B, Falanga A, Vannotti P, Fossati G, Semeraro N, Gordon SG (1986) Cancer procoagulant in human tumor cells: evidence from melanoma patients. *Cancer Res* 46: 6471
48. Falanga A, Alessio MG, Donati MB, Barbui T (1988) A new procoagulant in acute leukemia. *Blood* 71: 870–875
49. Gordon SG, Hashiba U, Poole MA, Cross BA, Falanga A (1985) A cysteine proteinase procoagulant from amnion-chorion. *Blood* 66: 1261
50. Buchanan MR, Dejana E, Cazenave J-P, Richardson M, Mustard JF, Hirsh J (1980) Differences in inhibition of PGI_2 production by aspirin in rabbit artery and vein segments. *Thromb Res* 20: 447–460
51. Dyerberg J, Bang HO (1979) Haemostatic function and platelet polyunsaturated fatty acids in Eskimos. *Lancet* II: 433–435
52. Knapp HR, Reilly IAG, Alessandrini P, FitzGerald GA (1986) In vivo indexes of platelet and vascular function during fish-oil administration in patients with atherosclerosis. *N Engl J Med* 314: 937–942
53. Grundy SM, Bonanome A (1987) Workshop on monounsaturated fatty acids. *Arteriosclerosis* 7: 644–648

Models of human renal disease

CARLA ZOJA, NORBERTO PERICO and GIUSEPPE REMUZZI
Institute for Pharmacological Research 'Mario Negri', Bergamo, Italy

Introduction

During the last few years exciting new insights into the mechanisms underlying the development of human renal diseases have been obtained from animal experiments. For the interpretation of the pathogenesis of membranous glomerulonephritis in man, important knowledge has been gained from the Heymann glomerulonephritis model in rats. Experimental studies enabled us to establish that interaction of antibodies with cell surface antigen results in antigen redistribution, immune complex aggregation and shedding, which are influenced by physiological forces of flow, filtration, and diffusion [1, 2]. Experimental models of chronic renal failure, particularly the renal mass ablation model in rats, provided a tool for understanding the characteristics of the deleterious intrarenal processes responsible for the progression of several human renal diseases to glomerulosclerosis and renal failure [3]. Several factors such as glomerular capillary hypertension and hyperperfusion, coagulation abnormalities, and alterations of lipid metabolism have been proposed as accounting for progressive glomerulosclerosis after nephrectomy [4–6]. The availability of experimental models of renal disease which closely mimic the human condition has greatly helped in defining therapeutic strategies such as dietary or pharmacological manipulations aimed at preventing or retarding the progression of kidney disease.

Here we will consider some experimental models of renal disease which have been of paramount importance in clarifying mechanisms of renal damage such as altered glomerular permselectivity to macromolecules and glomerular endothelial injury. The renal mass ablation model in rats is offered as an example for studying the factors involved in the inexorable progression of kidney disease which ultimately leads to end-stage renal failure. Finally, as a lesson from a clinical syndrome, we will analyze the role of atrial natriuretic peptide (ANP) in the fluid retention state which characterizes the edema in nephrotic syndrome, using the model of adriamycin nephrosis in rats.

S. Garattini (ed.), The Importance of Animal Experimentation for Safety and Biomedical Research, 111–123.

Mechanisms of renal damage

Altered glomerular permselectivity to proteins. Many studies have investigated the factors which, in the glomerular capillary wall, oppose the passage of circulating macromolecules into the urinary space. Studies with particulate tracers, cationic probes and immunohistochemical markers have now established that the glomerular capillary wall restricts the passage of circulating macromolecules by two major determinants: the size- and charge-selectivity properties of the glomerular basement membrane (GBM) [7–9]. The size-selective properties of GBM have been clearly demonstrated in animals with neutral dextrans of different molecular weight [10, 11], and the charge-selective properties have been documented employing ferritin with different isoelectric points [9, 12].

Chronic proteinuria in laboratory animals and humans often precedes the development of glomerular focal and segmental sclerosis, a lesion believed to be the main cause of progressive deteriorating renal function possibly due to hemodynamic changes in residual glomeruli. Advances in understanding the mechanisms of proteinuria and the subsequent development of focal and segmental sclerotic lesions derive from studies of two rat models: adriamycin (ADR) and puromycin aminonucleoside (PA) induced nephrosis. In both models the early phase of the disease is characterized by abnormal glomerular permeability to proteins, which precedes the development of glomerular sclerosis and renal function deterioration. In rats a single intravenous injection of ADR induces a nephrotic syndrome. The most widely employed model of ADR nephrosis employs a dose of 7.5 mg/kg of the drug [13]. However, recently it has been reported that a lower single dose (5 or 3 mg/kg) promotes chronic proteinuria in rats persisting several months [14]. The abnormal protein excretion begins a few days after the ADR injection and reaches its maximum after 14–16 days. Hypoalbuminemia and increased serum lipid levels are present. Histological examination of kidneys by light microscopy does not reveal any significant changes. Ultrastructural examination of the kidney shows extensive damage to the glomerular epithelial cells with diffuse swelling and foot process fusion. In the cytoplasm of proximal tubular cells protein reabsorption droplets are detected with casts in the distal tubules.

Puromycin nephrosis can be induced by a single injection (80 mg/kg) of aminonucleoside of puromycin (PA). Like in the ADR model proteinuria develops in a few days and reaches maximal values in 14–16 days. Animals also develop hypoalbuminemia and increases serum lipids [15]. Kidney ultrastructural alterations are very similar in both conditions [16]. However, at variance with the ADR model, animals given single i.v. injection of PA recover after four weeks of nephrotic syndrome [16]. Chronic and persistent proteinuria can be obtained in PA-treated animals only after repeated injections. ADR and PA nephrosis in rats have remarkable resemblances to human minimal change glomerulopathy as regards the morphological and clinical expression of the disease which is characterized by increased permeability to proteins, proteinuria, hypoalbuminemia, peripheral edema and hyperlipemia.

Factors involved in the altered glomerular capillary permeability to proteins in nephrotic syndrome are still unclear. It has been recently recognized that arachidonic acid metabolites may play a role in the development of proteinuria. Lianos *et al.* [17], in the rat model of nephrotoxic nephritis, found a linear correlation between proteinuria and the increase in glomerular thromboxane A2 (TxA2) synthesis.

In order to clarify a possible cause-effect relationship between proteinuria and increased renal TxA2, we studied the renal metabolism of AA in ADR nephrosis and found a significant increase of both glomerular production of TxB2, the stable breakdown product of TxA2, and urinary excretion of TxB2 [18]. No significant changes were found in the glomerular synthesis and urinary excretion of the other major AA metabolites formed through cyclooxygenase, namely 6-keto-PGF1_α, the stable breakdown product of PGI_2, and PGE_2. The increase in TxB2 was concomitant with the appearance of proteinuria and reached its maximum at the time of peak proteinuria. Administration of UK-38, 485, a selective TxA2 synthase inhibitor, to nephrotic animals significantly reduced the excessive renal TxA2 production and lowered proteinuria in all animals. This suggests that the mechanism of proteinuria, at least in this experimental model, depends on increased glomerular TxA2 synthesis which probably mediates an alteration in the glomerular barrier to proteins.

In the light of these observations in animals, the role of TxA2 as a possible mediator of proteinuria has now been investigated in chronic glomerulonephritis patients with and without nephrotic syndrome [19]. Increased urinary excretion of TxB2 has been reported in these patients. Of most interest is the recent observation that a TxA2 synthase inhibitor reduced the excessive urinary excretion of TxB2 and lowered urinary protein excretion in patients with minimal change nephrotic syndrome and that one of these patients, resistent to previous therapy, underwent remission with the TxA2-synthase inhibitor alone [20].

Besides pharmacological manipulation, urinary protein excretion in experimental nephrotic syndrome can be markedly influenced by changes in dietary protein intake. In rats with ADR nephrosis it has been reported that unlike animals fed a standard diet (20% protein), rats fed a low-protein diet (6%) neither developed proteinuria nor showed significant abnormalities of glomerular epithelial cells [21]. The effect of the low-protein diet did not appear to be the consequence of changes in renal blood flow and glomerular filtration rate. It has also been hypothesized that the protective effect of a low-protein diet could involve preservation of the permeability properties of the filtering membrane. Indeed the glomerular capillary normally impedes filtration of circulating macromolecules, acting as a size- and charge-selective barrier [7, 22]. Animal and human experiments have indicated that changes in virtual membrane pore radii or in the membrane negative charges [23–25] may alter glomerular selectivity for macromolecules allowing plasma proteins to cross the glomerular membrane and reach the urinary space. It is therefore conceivable that ADR induces proteinuria by altering one or both of these membrane filtering properties.

Conflicting data have been reported in ADR nephrosis as regards the nature of the glomerular sieving defect. Weening and Rennke [26], measuring the fractional clearance of anionic, native and cationic horseradish peroxidases in this model, found that the increased filtration of macromolecules was due to a great extent to a size-selectivity defect of the capillary wall, while charge-dependent permeability was unaltered. However, Bertolatus and coworkers [27] reported an almost complete loss of charge-dependent permselectivity, as indicated by comparable glomerular sieving coefficients for anionic and charge-modified neutral bovine serum albumin.

We have recently addressed the question of the nature of the altered glomerular permeability to macromolecules in ADR nephrosis [25]. Our results indicated that filtration of smaller neutral dextrans was comparable in proteinuric and normal animals, whereas the fractional clearance of larger dextran molecules (> 46 Å effective molecular radius) was increased in proteinuric animals, confirming a defect in size dependent selectivity in ADR nephrosis. Similarly, we found an increase in the fractional clearance of dextran sulfate (charged dextrans) molecules larger than 30 Å in molecular radius in ADR nephrotic rats. However the charge selectivity is not completely lost in animals with ADR nephrosis since, despite an increase in dextran sulfate fractional clearance in ADR rats, filtration of the charged molecules of 36 Å in effective molecular radius was still markedly restricted compared to the neutral molecules of comparable molecular radius.

These findings suggest that in ADR nephrosis a selective abnormality arises in both the size and charge restriction properties of the largest pores, which become less efficient in restricting macromolecule filtration, while the rest of the pore population is probably intact. Using a similar approach we found that a dietary regimen with low-protein intake in ADR nephrosis (6%) not only influenced the glomerular size selectivity, as indicated by a complete normalization of neutral dextran fractional clearance, but also influenced the charge-selective properties of the glomerular barrier [28]. Actually the charge-dependent selectivity was improved only for dextran sulfate radii greater than 36 Å. Therefore the beneficial effect of dietary protein restriction on glomerular permselectivity is the result of a complete preservation of size-selective function, while charge-dependent permselectivity is only partially restored.

Altogether these findings in the ADR nephrosis model have shed considerably more light on the mechanism by which low-protein feeding reduces proteinuria, lessens morphological alterations to the glomerular capillary wall and retards the progression of glomerular injury toward glomerulosclerosis in patients with chronic glomerulonephritis with or without nephrotic syndrome.

Vascular injury. Hemolytic uremic syndrome (HUS) and thrombotic thrombocytopenic purpura (TTP) are both characterized by thrombocytopenia, microangiopathic hemolytic anemia, renal disease and microthrombi occluding arterioles and capillaries of different organs [29–31]. Because of the simultaneous occurrence of thrombosis and microangiopathic anemia, the term 'thrombotic microangiopathy' (TMA) has been used to describe both syndromes [32]. The cause of microvascular thrombi in TMA is still debated. The recent demonstration of HUS in association with bacterial infections [33] and the finding of an *E. coli*-derived endotoxin (vero-cell verotoxin) in the stool of children with HUS support the possibility that certain strains of *E. coli* play a key role in the development of microvascular lesions [34, 35]. Moreover, evidence is available that besides bacterial products [36–38], antibodies or immune complexes [39] or certain drugs [40–42] are etiologic factors too in most cases of TMA.

The sequence of events leading to the microvascular changes following endotoxemia in humans and laboratory animals is ill-defined. Recently a model of continuous endotoxin infusion has been developed in the rabbit which induces a syndrome closely resembling human HUS [43]. We used this model to analyze the sequence of glomerular pathological changes occurring in the rabbit at various intervals after endotoxin infusion [44]. Rabbits were intravenously infused with endotoxin at a dose of 40 μg/kg/h for 5 hours. Endotoxin induced a significant drop in leukocyte and platelet counts in the peripheral blood and the animals developed anemia and renal failure. The biochemical changes were reversible, blood parameters returning to normal by 48 hours. Light microscopy showed marked polymorphonuclear cell infiltration in the glomerular capillary lumens as the prominent finding within 1 hour from the beginning of the infusion. At 5 hours fibrin deposits and thrombi were detected in most animals. These abnormalities were reversible. Electron microscopy detected endothelial damage a few minutes after the beginning of endotoxin infusion followed by leukocyte and platelet infiltration in glomerular capillaries. Fibrin appeared at 5 hours as free strands in the lumens or large clumps along the laminal surface of the endothelial layer. In more heavily damaged glomeruli fibrin had the appearance of capillary thrombi and was found under the endothelial cells. At 48 hours only mild endothelial damage remained, associated with a few polymorphonuclear cells in the glomerular capillary lumens.

The finding that polymorphonuclear cell infiltration follows endothelial damage and is only detected 1 hour from the beginning of endotoxin infusion suggests that a factor of endothelial origin is likely to be the signal for polymorphonuclear cell accumulation in glomeruli. The concomitant development of signs of leukocyte activation and renal damage suggests a cause and effect relationship between the two.

Since the tissue injury elicited by endotoxin may be largely mediated by tumor necrosis factor (TNF), a macrophage-derived polypeptide hormone [45, 46], we recently investigated whether TNF could directly induce glomerular damage [47]. We found that a 5-hour infusion of TNF to rabbits was associated with the development of glomerular changes, which included glomerular endothelial damage, polymorphonuclear cell accumulation in the capillary lumens and fibrin formation, very similar to those found in rabbits given endotoxin. These data provide further support to the concept that the deleterious effects of endotoxin in animals are mediated by TNF [48] and open new perspectives for microvascular thrombosis syndromes with maneuvers aimed at reducing TNF generation.

Mechanisms of progression of renal disease

Patients with moderate renal insufficiency almost invariably progress to end stage renal failure [3, 5]. This occurs even when common putative risk factors, such as hypertension and urinary tract infection, are excluded. These observations suggest that after a certain point the drop in nephron number leads to failure of the remaining units. The necessity of interrupting the progression of renal disease has stimulated the development of experimental models of chronic renal insufficiency and the investigation of the mechanism(s) responsible for the eventual destruction of the remaining nephrons.

As early as 1932 Chanutin and Ferris [49] observed that removal of 3/4 of the total renal mass in rats led to a slowly progressive deterioration in the function of the remaining nephrons, with significant proteinuria, progressive azotemia and glomerular sclerosis, as in progressive renal disease in humans. Chronic renal failure in rats can be obtained either by ligation of renal artery branches or by surgical removal of renal parenchyma [50, 51]. Subtotal ablation of renal mass leads to structural and functional hypertrophy of the remaining nephrons [52]. These changes are deleterious to the glomerular microcirculation and induce ultrastructural alterations including vacuolization of epithelial cells, deposition of osmophilic droplets in these cells and foot process fusion. These ultrastructural alterations lead to progressive hyalinization and eventual sclerosis of remnant glomeruli. Subtotal nephrectomy also leads to changes in the function of the remaining nephrons in rats which include an immediate elevation in single nephron GFR (hyperfiltration) as a result of increased intraglomerular capillary pressure and glomerular perfusion [5]. These glomerular hemodynamic changes lead to a compensatory increase in single nephron GFR of surviving glomeruli which alleviates the reduction in total GFR caused by the initiating injury.

Evidence that increased intraglomerular capillary pressure and glomerular perfusion initiate glomerular injury has been obtained in this extensive renal ablation model in rats. It has been suggested that maneuvers limiting the increase in glomerular capillary pressure and flow may retard the progressive sclerosis. Thus in rats with ablation of renal mass a low-protein diet which limits glomerular capillary pressure and flow was associated with much less proteinuria and glomerular injury developed more slowly than in animals with equivalent ablation of renal tissue fed a standard diet [50].

Recently it has been demonstrated that control of glomerular hypertension by pharmacological manipulation with an angiotensin I converting enzyme inhibitor, enalapril, limited glomerular injury in rats with renal ablation and this further supports the view that glomerular hemodynamic changes mediate progressive renal injury when nephron number is reduced [53]. The observation that converting enzyme inhibitors impede the progression of renal disease in rat models has raised the possibility that such therapy might have a place in human medicine. Unfortunately little information is available in humans as yet.

Vascular coagulation, with eventual thrombosis of glomerular capillaries, has also been suggested to have a role in glomerular injury following renal ablation [6]. Thus experimental studies have focussed on the possibility that prevention of blood coagulation might retard the development of progressive renal damage and hypertension in rats with renal mass reduction. Heparin and warfarin have proved effective in protecting rats with renal mass ablation from the development of glomerular sclerosis and in prolonging their survival [54, 55]. These therapies were associated not only with anticoagulation but also with significant lowering of systemic blood pressure.

The possibility that intraglomerular thrombosis and platelet aggregation play a role in the progression of renal disease in the remnant kidney model has been addressed by Purkerson *et al.* [56] who were able to reduce the severity of progressive renal disease in rats with renal mass ablation by using an inhibitor of thromboxane synthesis. This protection occurred despite an increase in GFR and RPF, that is, despite marked hyperfiltration. On the basis of these findings the authors suggested that factor(s) other than hemodynamics were responsible for progressive renal disease in this model. Moreover, since the TxA2 synthase inhibitor used in this study, besides preventing platelet aggregation and TxA2 formation, also lowered systemic blood pressure in these animals, the role of platelet TxA2 formation in the progression of renal damage to glomerular sclerosis in the renal mass ablation model remains to be clarified.

We have recently shown that ASA, at a dose fully suppressing platelet TxA2 formation but sparing renal cyclooxygenase, did not prevent progressive glomerular sclerosis in rats with remnant kidney [57]. These experiments appear to exclude that platelet TxA2 plays an important role in renal disease progression. However, TxA2 is just one of the many factors potentially released by activating platelets that may interfere with the progressive loss of renal function in remnant kidney. Therapeutic strategies aimed at retarding the process of progressive glomerular sclerosis based on drugs which block a wide spectrum of platelet reactions rather than on molecules which selectively block TxA2 biological activity merit further investigation.

Pathogenesis of edema in nephrotic syndrome: Lessons from animals

Edema, the clinical manifestation of an expanded interstitial fluid volume, is present in almost all patients with nephrotic syndrome at some time during the course of the disease. Swelling of the lower limbs or weight gain are the complaints that most often lead patients to seek medical advice. In any edematous state, progressive expansion of the extracellular fluid compartment ultimately requires concomitant retention of salt and water by the kidneys. The classic interpretation of a decrease in effective blood volume triggering renal sodium and water retention in edematous disorders, however, appears less germane to the nephrotic syndrome. Specifically, the traditional view of a decrease in intravascular volume secondary to proteinuria and hypoalbuminemia causing renal sodium and water retention in nephrotic syndrome [58] is not consistently applicable.

For example, several investigators have reported that some patients with nephrotic syndrome may actually have an increase in intravascular volume [59]. Moreover, despite adequate volume expansion, diuresis and natriuresis occurred in only half the treated nephrotic patients [60, 61]. These observations argue strongly in favor of an alternative explanation for edema in nephrotic syndrome, namely that sodium retention by the kidney is a primary event in response to intrarenal rather than systemic mechanisms.

Two recent studies of experimental nephrotic syndrome induced by intravenous injection of PA, a model of minimal change nephropathy, have produced clear evidence of renal sodium retention from local intrarenal cause(s) [62, 63]. These elegant studies have yielded important data that have greatly clarified our understanding of how nephrotic patients with edema may develop the apparently confusing picture of normal blood volume or hypervolemia. In this experimental model, only one kidney of each animal was perfused with PA so that unilateral proteinuria was produced and hypoalbuminemia did not develop. Sodium excretion was normal or high from the nonperfused control kidney, but was significantly reduced from the PA-perfused, proteinuric kidneys at a time when systemic plasma protein concentration, and presumably blood volume, was normal. This evidence clearly suggests that the primary cause of the sodium retention resides in the kidneys.

A detailed micropuncture study of the unilateral nephrotic kidney further demonstrated that sodium retention depends upon changes in tubular function beyond the distal convolution [62], although the cause of the retention is still unknown. The recent discovery [64] of the natriuretic effect of atrial peptides (ANP) and of their possible role in volume regulation [65] raises the question of their involvement in the nephrotic syndrome. Three alternative possibilities are that the atrial content of ANP is reduced or its secretion is impaired in the nephrotic syndrome or that the nephrotic kidney is unresponsive to ANP. We have found that atrial extracts from rats with ADR nephrosis, an experimental model in which the clinical and morphological expression of the disease resembles minimal change nephropathy in humans [13], when injected in control rats, induced a diuretic and natriuretic response comparable with that of atrial extracts from normal rats [66]. Thus the atrial content of ANP in nephrotic rats must be similar to that of control animals.

Atrial release from the heart can be induced by a number of stimuli including atrial distension, saline expansion and an increase in central vascular volume [67–69]. Testing the ability of nephrotic rats to secrete ANP in response to volume expansion, Keeler and coworkers [70] found no difference in secretory response of ANP in PA-treated rats and untreated rats and concluded that in nephrotic rats failure to secrete ANP does not occur.

To establish whether the kidney in nephrotic syndromes is unresponsive to ANP we infused atrial extract or synthetic ANP into ADR nephrotic rats [66]. The diuretic and natriuretic response to ANP was markedly attenuated in nephrotic animals as compared to control rats. Since the blunted diuretic and natriuretic response to ANP occurred despite a comparable percentage rise in glomerular filtration rate, it is suggested that the defect lies in more distal segments of the nephron. The findings obtained experimentally in animals have been confirmed in humans by Hricik *et al.* [71]. Studying the effect of human ANP infusion in patients with nephrotic syndrome or cirrhosis with ascites, they found only a mild increase in fractional excretion of sodium as compared to the marked increase observed after furosemide. This latter observation reinforces the hypothesis that the retention of salt and water by the kidneys in nephrotic syndrome reflects a specific abnormal resistance of the nephrotic kidney to ANP not shared with other diuretics [72].

We have recently investigated whether the abnormal renal response to ANP is due to systemic or intrarenal changes using a unilateral model of ADR-induced proteinuria [73]. The diuretic and natriuretic response of the infusion of synthetic ANP was markedly blunted in the kidney exposed to ADR but not in the contralateral one. This occurred without detectable abnormalities in the glomerular response to ANP in terms of GFR. Thus intrarenal unresponsiveness to ANP may be the key factor in the sodium retaining state which characterizes edema in the nephrotic syndrome. The mechanism(s) underlying the abnormal renal response to ANP is open to speculation. Further investigations are necessary to establish whether ANP receptors in the kidneys of nephrotic rats have an altered sensitivity to ANP, as a consequence of a decrease in receptor density or affinity.

References

1. Kerjaschki D, Miettinen A, Farquhar MG (1987) Initial events in the formation of immune deposits in Passive Heymann Nephritis. gp330-anti-gp330 immune complexes form in epithelial coated pits and rapidly become attached to the glomerular basement membrane. *J Exp Med* 166: 109–28
2. Andres G, Brentjens JR, Caldwell PRB, Camussi G, Matsuo S (1986) Biology of disease. Formation of immune deposits and disease. *Lab Invest* 55: 510–20
3. Klahr S, Schreiner G, Ichikawa I (1988) The progression of renal disease. *N Engl J Med* 318: 1657–66
4. Hostetter TH, Olson JL, Rennke HG, Venkatachalam MA, Brenner BM (1981) Hyperfiltration in remnant nephrons: a potentially adverse response to renal ablation. *Am J Physiol* 241: F85–F93
5. Anderson S, Meyer TW, Brenner BM (1985) The role of hemodynamic factors in the initiation and progression of renal disease. *J Urol* 133: 310–315
6. Klahr S, Heifets M, Purkerson ML (1986) The influence of anticoagulation on the progression

of experimental renal disease. In: Mitch WE, Brenner BM, Stein JH (Eds) *The progressive nature of renal disease*. New York: Churchill Livingstone pp 45–64

7. Brenner BM, Hostetter TH, Humes HD (1978) Molecular basis of proteinuria of glomerular origin. *N Engl J Med* 298: 826–833
8. Farquhar MG (1981) The glomerular basement membrane – a selective macromolecular filter. In: Hay ED (Ed) *The Cell Biology of the Extracellular Matrix*. New York: Plenum Press p 335
9. Rennke HG, Cotran RS, Venkatachalam MA (1975) Role of molecular charge in glomerular permeability. Tracer studies with cationized ferritin. *J Cell Biol* 67: 638–646
10. Chang RLS, Ueki IF, Troy JL, Deen WM, Robertson CR, Brenner BM (1975) Permselectivity of glomerular capillary wall to macromolecules. II. Experimental studies in rats using neutral dextran. *Biophys J* 15: 887–906
11. Rennke HG, Venkatachalam MA, Patel Y (1979) Glomerular permeability of macromolecules: effect of molecular configuration on the fractional clearance of uncharged dextran and neutral horseradish peroxidase in the rat. *J Clin Invest* 63: 713–726
12. Rennke HG, Venkatachalam MA (1977) Glomerular permeability: in vivo tracer studies with polyanionic and polycationic ferritins. *Kidney Int* 11: 44–53
13. Bertani T, Poggi A, Pozzoni R, Delaini F, Sacchi G, Thoua Y, Mecca G, Remuzzi G, Donati MB (1982) Adriamycin-induced nephrotic syndrome in rats. Sequence of pathologic events. *Lab Invest* 46: 16–23
14. Bertani T, Rocchi G, Sacchi G, Mecca G, Remuzzi G (1986) Adriamycin-induced glomerulosclerosis in the rat. *Am J Kidney Diseases* 7: 12–19
15. Grond J, Weening JJ, Elema JD (1984) Glomerular sclerosis in nephrotic rats. Comparison of the long-term effects of adriamycin and aminonucleoside. *Lab Invest* 51: 277–285
16. Ryan GB, Karnovsky MJ (1975) An ultrastructural study of the mechanisms of proteinuria in aminonucleoside nephrosis. *Kidney Int* 8: 219–232
17. Lianos EA, Andres GA, Dunn MJ (1983) Glomerular prostaglandin and thromboxane synthesis in rat nephrotoxic serum nephritis. Effects on renal hemodynamics. *J Clin Invest* 72: 1439–1448
18. Remuzzi G, Imberti L, Rossini M, Morelli C, Carminati C, Cattaneo GM, Bertani T (1985) Increased glomerular thromboxane synthesis as a possible cause of proteinuria in experimental nephrosis. *J Clin Invest* 75: 94–101
19. Niwa T, Maeda K, Shibata M (1987) Urinary prostaglandins and thromboxane in patients with chronic glomerulonephritis. *Nephron* 46: 281–288
20. Niwa T, Ozawa Y, Nomura T, Maeda K, Shibata M (1987) Thromboxane A2 metabolism and clinical effects of selective thromboxane A2 synthetase inhibitor in chronic glomerulonephritis. Xth International Congress of Nephrology. London, July 26–31, p 24
21. Remuzzi G, Zoja C, Remuzzi A, Rossini M, Battaglia C, Broggini M, Bertani T (1985) Low-protein diet prevents glomerular damage in adriamycin-treated rats. *Kidney Int* 28: 21–27
22. Brenner BM, Bohrer MP, Baylis C, Deen WM (1977) Determinants of glomerular permselectivity: insights derived from observations *in vivo*. *Kidney Int* 12: 229–37
23. Deen WM, Bridges CR, Brenner BM, Myers BD (1985) Heteroporous model of glomerular size selectivity: application to normal and nephrotic humans. *Am J Physiol* 249 (Renal Fluid Electrolyte Physiol 18): F364–F389
24. Deen WM, Satvat B (1981) Determinants of the glomerular filtration of proteins. *Am J Physiol* 241 (10): F162–F170
25. Remuzzi A, Battaglia C, Rossi L, Zoja C, Remuzzi G (1987) Glomerular size-selectivity in nephrotic rats exposed to diets with different protein content. *Am J Physiol* 253: F318–F327
26. Weening JJ, Rennke HG (1983) Glomerular permeability and polyanion in adriamycin nephrosis in the rat. *Kidney Int* 24: 152–159
27. Bertolatus JA, Hunsicker LG (1985) Glomerular sieving of anionic and neutral bovine albumins in proteinuric rats. *Kidney Int* 28: 467–76

28. Remuzzi A, Battaglia C, Remuzzi G (1988) Effect of low-protein diet on size and charge permeability in experimental nephrosis. [Abstr] In: *21st Annual Meeting of the American Society of Nephrology*. December 11–14
29. Fong JSC, de Chadarevian J-P, Kaplan BS (1982) Hemolytic-uremic syndrome. Current concepts and management. *Ped Clin North Am* 29: 835–56
30. Bukowski RM (1982) Thrombotic thrombocytopenic purpura: A review. In: Spaet TH (Ed), *Progress in Hemostasis and Thrombosis*. New York: Grune & Stratton, pp 287–337
31. Remuzzi G (1987) HUS and TTP: Variable expression of a single entity. *Kidney Int* 32: 292–308
32. Rossi EC, Carone FA, del Greco F (1980) Hemolytic-uremic syndrome and platelet-endothelial interactions. In: Remuzzi G, Mecca G, de Gaetano G (Eds). *Hemostasis, Prostaglandins and Renal Disease*. New York: Raven Press, pp 321–329
33. Koster F, Levin J, Walker L, Tung KSK, Gilman RH, Rahaman MM, Majid MA, Islam S, Williams RC (1978) Hemolytic-uremic syndrome after shigellosis: relation to endotoxemia and circulating immune complexes. *N Engl J Med* 298: 927–933
34. Karmali MA, Steele BT, Petric M, Lim C (1983) Sporadic cases of haemolytic-uraemic syndrome associated with faecal cytotoxin and cytotoxin-producing Escherichia coli in stools. *Lancet* 1: 619–620
35. Karmali MA, Petric M, Lim C, Fleming PC, Arbus GS, Lior H (1985) The association between idiopathic hemolytic uremic syndrome and infection by verotoxin-producing Escherichia coli. *J Infect Dis* 151: 775–782
36. Amorosi EL, Ultmann JE (1966) Thrombotic Thrombocytopenic Purpura: Report of 16 cases and review of the literature. *Medicine (Baltimore)* 45: 139–159
37. Morrison DM, Tyrrel DLJ, Jewell LD (1986) Colonic biopsy in verotoxin-induced hemorrhagic colitis and thrombotic thrombocytopenic purpura (TTP). *Am J Clin Pathol* 86: 108–112
38. Morton AR, Yu R, Waldek S, Holems AM, Craig A, Mundy K (1985) Campylobacter induced thrombotic thrombocytopenic purpura. *Lancet* 2: 1133–1134
39. Wall RT, Harker LA (1980) The endothelium and thrombosis. *Ann Rev Med* 31: 361–371
40. Brown CG, Clarkson AP, Robson JS, Cameron JS, Thomson D, Ogg CS (1973) Haemolytic-uraemic syndrome in women taking oral contraceptives. *Lancet* 1: 1479–1481
41. Shulman H, Striker G, Deeg HJ, Kennedy M, Storb R, Thomas ED (1981) Nephrotoxicity of Cyclosporin A after allogeneic marrow transplantation: glomerular thrombosis and tubular injury. *N Engl J Med* 305: 1392–1395
42. Lyman NW, Michaelson R, Viscuso RL, Winn R, Mulgaonakar S, Jacobs MG (1983) Mitomycin-induced hemolytic uremic syndrome. Successful treatment with corticosteroids and intense plasma exchange. *Arch Intern Med* 143: 1617–1618
43. Vedanarayanan VV, Kaplan BS, Fong JSC (1987) Neutrophil function in an experimental model of hemolytic uremic syndrome. *Pediatr Res* 21: 252–256
44. Bertani T, Abbate M, Zoja C, Corna D, Remuzzi G. Sequence of glomerular changes in an experimental model of hemolytic uremic syndrome due to endotoxemia (submitted for publication)
45. Old LJ: Tumor necrosis factor (TNF) (1985) *Science* 230: 630–632
46. Aggarwal BB, Kohr WJ, Hass PE, Moffat B, Spencer SA, Henzel WJ, Bringman TS, Nedwin GE, Goeddel DV, Harkins RN (1985) Human tumor necrosis factor. Production, purification and characterization. *J Biol Chem* 260: 2345–2354
47. Bertani T, Abbate M, Zoja C, Corna D, Perico N, Ghezzi P, Remuzzi G. Tumor necrosis factor (TNF) induces glomerular damage in the rabbit. *Am J Pathol* (in press)
48. Beutler B, Milsark IW, Cerami AC (1985) Passive immunization against cachectin-tumor necrosis factor protects mice from lethal effect of endotoxin. *Science* 869–871
49. Chanutin A, Ferris EB Jr (1932) Experimental renal insufficiency produced by partial nephrectomy. I. Control diet. *Arch Intern Med* 49: 767–787
50. Olson JL, Hostetter TH, Rennke HG, Brenner BM, Venkatachalam MA (1982) Altered glomerular permselectivity and progressive sclerosis following extreme ablation of renal mass.

Kidney Int 22: 112–126
51. Ormrod D, Miller T (1980) Experimental uremia. Description of a model producing varying degrees of stable uremia. *Nephron* 26: 249–254
52. Shimamura T, Morrison AB (1975) A progressive glomerulosclerosis occurring in partial fix-sixths nephrectomized rats. *Am J Pathol* 79: 95–106
53. Anderson S, Rennke HG, Brenner BM (1986) Therapeutic advantage of converting enzyme inhibitors in arresting progressive renal disease associated with systemic hypertension in the rat. *J Clin Invest* 77: 1993–2000
54. Purkerson ML, Joist JH, Greenberg JM, Kay D, Hoffsten PE, Klahr S (1982) Inhibition by anticoagulant drugs of the progressive hypertension and uremia associated with renal infarction in rats. *Thromb Res* 26: 227–240
55. Olson JL (1984) Role of heparin as a protective agent following reduction of renal mass. *Kidney Int* 25: 376–382
56. Purkerson ML, Joist JH, Yates J, Valdes A, Morrison A, Klahr S (1985) Inhibition of thromboxane synthesis ameliorates the progressive kidney disease of rats with subtotal renal ablation. *Proc Natl Acad Sci* 82: 193–197
57. Zoja C, Benigni A, Livio M, Bergamelli A, Orisio S, Abbate M, Bertani T, Remuzzi G. Selective inhibition of platelet thromboxane generation with low-dose aspirin does not protect rats with reduced renal mass from the development of progressive disease (submitted for publication)
58. Bernard D-B, Alexander EA (1979) Edema formation in the nephrotic syndrome: Pathophysiologic mechanisms. *Cardiovasc Med* 4: 605–625
59. Dorhout Mees EJ, Geers AB, Koomans HA (1984) Blood volume and sodium retention in the nephrotic syndrome: A controversial pathophysiology concept. *Nephron* 36: 201–211
60. Luetscher JA, Hall AD, Kremer VL (1950) Treatment of nephrosis with concentrated human serum albumin. II. Effects on renal function and on excretion of water and some electrolytes. *J Clin Invest* 29: 896–905
61. Orloff J, Welt LG, Stowe L (1950) The effects of concentrated salt-poor albumin on the metabolism and excretion of water and electrolytes in nephrosis and toxemia of pregnancy. *J Clin Invest* 29: 770–780
62. Ichikawa I, Rennke HG, Hoyer JR, Badr KF, Schor N, Troy JL, Lechene CP, Brenner BM (1983) Role for intrarenal mechanisms in the impaired salt excretion of experimental nephrotic syndrome. *J Clin Invest* 71: 91–103
63. Chandra M, Hoyer JR, Lewy JE (1981) Renal function in rats with unilateral proteinuria produced by renal perfusion with aminonucleoside. *Pediatr Res* 15: 340–344
64. De Bold AJ, Borenstein BH, Veress AT, Sonnenberg A (1981) A rapid and potent natriuretic response to intravenous injection of atrial myocardial extract in rats. *Life Sci* 28: 89–94
65. Ballerman BJ, Brenner BM (1985) Biologically active atrial peptides. *J Clin Invest* 76: 2041–2408
66. Perico N, Delaini F, Lupini C, Remuzzi G (1987) Renal response to atrial peptides is reduced in experimental nephrosis. *Am J Physiol* 252: F654–F660
67. Dietz JR (1984) Release of natriuretic factor from rat heart-lung preparation by atrial distension. *Am J Physiol* 247: R1093–R1096
68. Salazar FJ, Romero JC, Burnett JC Jr, Schryver S, Granger JP (1986) Atrial natriuretic peptide levels during acute and chronic saline loading in conscious dogs. *Am J Physiol* 251: R499–R503
69. Miki K, Hajduczok G, Klocke MR, Kransey JA, Hong SK, De Bold AJ (1986) Atrial natriuretic factor and renal function during head-out water immersion in conscious dogs. *Am J Physiol* 251: R1000–R1008
70. Keeler R, Feuchuk D, Wilson N (1987) Atrial peptides and the renal response to hypervolemia in nephrotic rats. *Can J Physiol Pharmacol* 65: 2071–2075
71. Hricik DE, Appel RG, Simonson MJ, Green J, Smith R, Dunn MJ (1987) Effects of human atrial natriuretic factor (ANF) in patients with nephrotic syndrome (NS) and cirrhosis with ascites (CA). [Abstr] *Kidney Int* 31 (1): 273

72. Hildebrandt DA, Banks RD (1988) Effect of atrial natriuretic factor on renal function in rats with nephrotic syndrome. *Am J Physiol* 254: F210–F216
73. Delaini F, Perico N, Lupini C, Tagliaferri M, Remuzzi G (1988) Increased plasma volume and atrial natriuretic peptide (ANP) but reduced diuresis for an intrarenal defect in adriamycin (ADR)-induced nephrotic syndrome (ADR). [Abstr] *Kidney Int* 33 (1): 261

The necessity of animal experimentation in tumor immunology

GUIDO FORNI, PATRIZIA CARETTO, PAOLA FERRAIORNI, MARIA CARLA BOSCO and MIRELLA GIOVARELLI
Institute of Microbiology, University of Turin, Turin, Italy

Introduction

The world is overcrowded with human beings often pressed against one another or standing in queues. Their lives are spent in a struggle to dominate small spaces in which to act, or tiny sections of a street in which to move within an environment made unpleasant by noise, odeurs and waste generated by other human beings. Because of these continuous, forced close encounters, the bonds between them as members of the same species slacken and the pleasure of finding other humans and sharing things with them vanishes. By contrast, contact with almost any other animal species is becoming a rare event. Animals are now precious, protected and often beloved survivors. Thus, step by step man are turning out to be emotionally more disturbed by the sufferings of animals than by the common, unpleasant sufferings of other man.

Every scientist thus has a personal and social duty to evaluate and decide whether animal experimentation is necessary for the endeavors of science. He has to weigh on imaginary scales the suffering imposed to the animals and the potential benefits. In the field of immunology, tumor immunology in particular, the potential benefits expected not only for the human species but for the upper vertebrates in general appear to be high.

Complexity of the immune system

The immune system is the second largest body apparatus. It consists of many cell populations such as granulocytes, macrophages and lymphocytes, each of which can be further subdivided in sub-populations of cells designed to perform particular functions. However, the functions of the immune system are not carried out by the single cells, but are induced and regulated through cooperation between numerous and distinct leukocytes. This cell-cell communication takes place through interactions with particular molecules expressed on the membrane of the partner cell and the secretion of soluble factors,

S. Garattini (ed.), The Importance of Animal Experimentation for Safety and Biomedical Research, 125–132.

called lymphokines and monokines [1–3]. As suggested by their name, which comes from the Greek verb kinein meaning to move the activity of these molecules is to shift predetermined populations of leukocytes into gear for operation.

The cell-cell interaction phase is highly specific since the cells gather together only if they reciprocally recognize specific molecular conformations on the membrane. Once the cell-cell conjugate is formed, a polarized secretion of mono-lymphokines takes place primarily over the small area of the membrane in which the two cells are in contact [3]. Paracrine (or even autocrine) secretion of mono-lymphokines may also serve as a less efficient system of recruiting nearby bystander leukocytes in the reaction. Distinct leukocytes elicit distinct response patterns following the release of distinct lymphokine cocktails [4].

As the immune system is a real network of multiple and highly interactive reaction mechanisms, modification of a single mesh affects the equilibrium of the whole system.

Computer and mathematical modelling

Reproduction or prediction of the outcome of immunological functions and manipulation by mathematical models has long been a dream. Computers are instrumental to this goal. Interesting models have been proposed and are currently elaborated [5]. However, since the immune system is so multifactorial and interactive realistic models are still too complicated to build. Moreover, ironically, the model becomes more accurate as our knowledge of basic immune mechanisms becomes larger. This means that more data must be provided by *in vitro* and *in vivo* experiments. Computer aided data processing is currently used in their interpretation.

Problems associated with *in vitro* experimentation

How are we to study such a complex interactive system? The reductionistic method calls for fragmentation of the immune system and study of its simple mechanisms and interactions. This is currently a mainstream method in immunological research. Cells and organs are taken away from the body, dissected, the cells fractionated and studied *in vitro*. This means that the cells are put in an environment that reproduces a few of the critical features of the body. They are nourished by artificially made media, heated and made to breathe in sophisticated incubators. In this way, they often survive so happily that they reproduce and perform a few of their activities. A single cell can even be isolated and persuaded to form a large progeny - a clone - of cells identical to the parent. This achievement is important to get enough homogeneous material (cells, membranes, nucleic acids...) to work with at functional, biochemical and molecular level.

By adding distinct stimuli to the culture, functional and molecular study is possible on the reactions elicited. Thus *in vitro* methods do give information and biological tools of crucial importance.

What is the difficulty, then? The *in vitro* environment can lead to over-emphasis - or under-assessment - of the relevance of some cell functions, mainly those recruiting numerous cell types. *In vitro* studies have not the prospective dimension. The analysis may be accurate but the tissue analyzed may be irrelevant, or may even not take place *in vivo*. The biological perspective can only be acquired by comparison of *in vitro* data with the *in vivo* situation.

Biological data become important only when they are not too influenced by a peculiar experimental situation. In order to start solving a problem, phenomenology and variability must be reduced as far as possible. Thus for many *in vitro* studies animals must be homogeneous as far as age, sex and genetic background are concerned. So animals are again directly involved, even in this kind of experimentation. Their suffering, however, is limited to a quick death. In most cases, only after a clear picture stems from these *in vitro* animal experimentations can the studies be extended to humans. But using human cells, the problem may become mixed up and the results inconstant because the donors are so ill-matched. Moreover, the studies have to be confined to blood cells, since it is rare to have access to fresh and normal spleen, lymph node or liver cells.

Ex vivo experiments

In vitro experiments are generally the more informative the fresher the cells involved in the experiments. Clones of cells established for a long time *in vitro* can provide very important information but it may be a misrepresentation of the real situation *in vivo*. Moreover, the need to use animals becomes more cogent if one has to evaluate a pathological condition or the effects of immunological treatment. Here, one needs both a normal control and a treated animal as cell donors. The analytical phase of the experiments may then be fully run *in vitro* but the real value of the data depends on close matching of the treated and control animals. A good biological perspective can be established by reference to the control and the pattern of change during the course of the disease or treatment. *Ex vivo* experiments thus provide important information, but require many variously treated animals.

This approach can be used in man. However, matching normal and untreated donors is exceedingly difficult and large series of data are needed to smooth out the differences between each individual donor. Moreover, it is currently considered unethical or even criminal to expose human volunteers to treatments that have not been fully tested in animals.

This issue, however, is linked to ethical values and intraspecies loyalty.

In vivo data: Trustworthiness and infidelity

By performing experiments on living animals, the efficacy of a treatment can be determined by evaluating the animal's survival and quality of life after a microbial or neoplastic challenge. Integration of the *in vivo*, *ex vivo* and *in vitro* findings will give a picture of the biological event studied. *In vitro* and *ex vivo* findings acquire a biological perspective when it can be shown that their modulation is causally related to better or longer survival. Moreover, by comparing the effects on mice of different genetic background it is possible to see to what extent the data apply on a general scale. In this sense, *in vivo veritas* is indisputable.

However, in most cases, the immune experiment done on animals is a model of a particular immunotherapy to be employed in humans. How far does the model represent the clinical situation? The question is inherent to any model. However, here it is more impelling as on the other side of the scales there are not only high costs and time, but particularly the suffering of living things.

Animal models in tumor immunology

Whilst in most immunological experiments animal models represent the human situation closely, in tumor immunology this problem is particularly complex. Immune tumor-host relationships are exceedingly intricate as the connatural and adaptive complexity of the immune system is added to the particular features of neoplastic cells and their progression [6].

The use of large groups of homogenous inbred rodents carrying immunogenic syngeneic tumors is instrumental both to tease apart the rules of this relationship and to assess the biological utility of immunomodulatory manoeuvres. Most of the information currently available on the features of tumor-host relationships and on the possibility of hampering neoplastic growth by immunological procedures are based on data obtained from animal experimentation [7]. In many cases, the data have been obtained using very immunogenic tumors which are, however, rare in nature [8]. These models do not present a realistic picture of human tumors, nor do they seek to do so. Rather, they serve to provide basic information. This is made possible by reducing the complex problem to simpler models in which some features of the situation they reflect are deliberately ignored. The use of highly immunogenic tumors in these studies is fully justified by the fact that currently we still have only a vage idea of the cell mechanisms involved in immune resistance to tumors [9].

Of course, the use of models can be dangerous. Some biological functions that appear to be crucial to a simplified system may loose their importance or take on a different meaning in more complex systems. The fact that it is a model, not the real situation, that is being studied may be forgotten.

The desperate need for tumor immunology

If the understanding and manipulation of the immune system appears very complex, why is so much effort being diverted to using immunological mechanisms in the control of tumors? The answer is tragically simple: the overall incidence of tumors is rising but gains in survival time of cancer patients and reductions of cancer death rates are marginal. Of those diagnosed with cancer, only half will be alive in five years time [10]. Surgery, radiotherapy and chemiotherapy are improving continuously, but there seems little to support the hope of major breakthroughs. Tumor immunology, on the other hand, may represent a completely new therapeutic approach. By itself, or integrated with conventional management, immunological manoeuvres may serve as a fresh start for cancer treatment [11].

Monoclonal antibodies are currently an important tool for early and accurate diagnosis of neoplasia. Soon they may become an important therapeutic instrument [12]. Several lymphokines are theurapeutic tools, as they have selective antiproliferative activity, are able to force tumor cells to differentiate to a non-neoplastic stage, enhance the immune recognition of tumor cells and elicit cytotoxic lymphocytes able to kill tumor cells discriminatingly [13].

Monoclonal antibodies are produced in animals. Monoclonal antibodies and lymphokines must be studied in pre-clinical animal models in order to arrange pilot clinical studies.

New preclinical models

The cloning of mono-lymphokine genes and their subsequent production in amounts large enough to be used in clinical practice are one of the most winning developments of cellular immunology. These molecules constitute a hormone-like communication code within the cells of the immune system, on which the regulation of intensity and duration of the activities induced by triggering signals depend. Lymphokines are thus a focal point in investigations on cell-mediated immunotherapy of tumors, since they make it possible to hark back to old anti-tumor strategies by exploiting their tremendous potentiality [2, 11, 13].

In effect, lymphokines appear capable to removing a few of the long-standing barriers that limit the clinical applicability of cell-mediated tumor immunotherapy, such as the difficulty of obtaining large numbers of specifically sensitized lymphocytes for use *in vivo*. Continuous cell lines of cytotoxic lymphocytes reactive against tumor-associated antigens have been maintained and expanded by using culture medium supplemented with one lymphokine (interleukin-2, IL-2). These expanded populations maintain their ability to kill tumor cells when injected *in vivo* and their survival can be prolonged by systematic injections of exogenous IL-2 [14]. In addition, the presence of IL-2 permits tumor recognition and the generation of a complex immune reaction by otherwise non-immunogenic tumor cells [15].

The data obtained in several *in vivo* models with mice bearing micrometastases and primary tumors with IL-2 activated cytotoxic lymphocytes and with IL-2 alone injected peritumorally and perilymphatically have led to the establishment of new treatment protocols for human cancer [16, 17]. In this case, the murine models were - and still are - instrumental for setting up new clinical strategies, since there is close parallelism between animal and clinical data [14–17].

The peculiarity of some human neoplasms, however, cannot be studied on conventional animal models, since we do not know yet of what the peculiarity consists. In effect, certain human tumors are particularly sensitive to certain immunological treatments (e.g. hairy cell leukemia to interferons; renal car cinoma to cytolytic activity of lymphokine-activated killer cells) [18]. Direct study on human patients, on the other hand, is extremely slow, difficult, often impossible or not justifiable, since it would be clinical experimentation on a purely empirical basis.

A possible approach is to use human tumors made to grow in immunosuppressed rodents. Nude mice (nu/nu) are mice whose lack of hair gives them a pink color. They have a rudimentary thymus consisting of fibroid tissue virtually devoid of lymphocytes. These animals have poor cellular immunoreactivity and are very prone to microbial infections. However, when maintained in a sterile environment they are as long-lived as conventional euthymic mice [19]. Human hemopoietic neoplasms do not grow in nude mice. By contrast, several fresh human lymphomas and leukemias grow in splenectomized, sublethally irradiated mice, which receive further injections of antibody that abolish their natural cell reactivity (SIA-nu/nu mice). Human leukemic cells maintain most of their structural and immunological features when injected in SIA-nu/nu mice. In many cases, the leukemic cells not only grow as solid tumors, but can also spread to the lymphoid tissues and reproduce several of the features and complications of the human disease [20].

The use of SIA-nu/nu mice for growing human neoplasms, and their repopulation with selected sets of human leukocytes constitute a new experimental system. Primary and metastatic solid and lymphoid tumors can be studied. Differentiation and the modulation of tumor progression and metastatic spread by various cytokines can be evaluated. Mono- and lymphokine modulation of the reactivity of human cells against human tumors can be analyzed in detail.

Of course these are models, and in a few respects very artificial ones. However, the data obtained from models of this kind can be very informative and constitute important guidelines for setting up rational pilot experimentation with cancer patients.

What are on the two sides of the scales?

The scales weigh up rational hope for a large population of human beings suffering and dying of cancer [7, 11–18] against a similar suffering in an even larger rodent population. Since, unfortunately, alternatives are not available for the realistic evaluation of immunological manoeuvres, the choice of using animals for further studies in tumor immunology is simple and clear for those who are familiar with the cruelty of cancer and who spend their life fighting it. The ones who disagree, honestly, without hiding behind dreams of currently inexistent alternative methods, are making a terrible choice. When this choice is not due to plain superficiality, it appears to us to be horribly cruel, as it leads to further rupture of the bonds of sympathy between members of the human species.

Acknowledgements

We thank Dr J. Iliffe for careful review of the manuscript. This paper was supported by grants from Prog. Ric. Finaliz. Regione Piemonte and the Italian Association for Cancer Research (AIRC).

References

1. Mitchison NA (1980) Regulation of the immune response to cell surface antigens. In: B Pernis and HJ Vogel (Eds) *Regulatory T lymphocytes*, Academic Press, New York, pp 147–157
2. Smith KA (1984) Interleukin 2. *Ann Rev Immunol* 2: 319–327
3. Janeway CA, Bottomly K, Horowitz J, Kaye J, Jones B, Tite J (1985) Modes of cell-cell communication in the immune system. *J Immunol* 135: 739s–742s
4. Mossman TR, Cherwinski H, Bond MW, Giedlin MA, Coffman RL (1986) Two types of murine helper T cell line. I. Definition according the profiles of lymphokine activity and secreted proteins. *J Immunol* 129: 2337–2341
5. Weiler E, Adam G, Schuler W, Weiler IJ (1976): Clonal selection and network regulation. In: F Melchers and K Rajewsky (Eds) *The immune system*, Springer Verlag, Berlin, pp 267–276
6. Forni G, Varesio L, Giovarelli M, Cavallo G. Dynamic state of spontaneous immune reactivity towards a mammary adenocarcinoma. In: Spreafico and Arnon (Eds) *Tumor antigens and their specific immune response*, Academic Press, pp 167–192
7. Herberman RB (1983) Animal tumor models and their relevance to human tumor immunology. *J Biol Resp Modif* 2: 39–46
8. Hewitt HB (1982) Animal tumor models for tumor immunology. *J Biol Resp Modif* 1: 107–119
9. Forni G, Santoni A (1984) Immunogenicity of non-immunogenic tumors. *J Biol Resp Modif* 3: 128–131
10. Rawlins RJ (1988) Editorial. *Molec Biotherapy* 1: 2–2
11. Oldham RK (1986) Biotherapy: General Principles. In: Oldham RK (Ed) *Principles of cancer biotherapy*. Raven Press, New York, pp 1–20
12. Dillman RO (1984) Monoclonal antibodies in the treatment of cancer. *CRC Crit Rv Hematol*

Oncol 1: 357–386

13. Forni G, Giovarelli, M (1987) Tumor immunotherapy with interleukin-2 and leukocytes. In: W Den Otter and EJ Ruitenberg (Eds) *Tumor Immunology-Mechanisms, Diagnosis, Therapy*. Elsevier Science Publishers BV, pp 265–273
14. Mule' JJ, Shu S, Schwarz SL, Rosenberg SA (1984) Adoptive immunotherapy of established pulmonary metastases with LAK cells and recombinant interleukin-2. *Science* 225: 1487–1490
15. Forni G, Giovarelli M, Santoni A, Modesti A and Forni M (1987) Interleukin 2 activated tumor inhibition 'in vivo' depends on the systemic involvement of host immunoreactivity. *J Immunol* 138: 4033–4039
16. Rosenberg SA, Lotze MT, Muul LM, Chang AE, Avis FP, Leitman S, Linehan WM, Robertson CN, Lee RE, Rubin JJT, Seipp CA, Simpson CG, White DE (1987) A progress report on the treatment of 157 patients with advanced cancer using lymphokine-activated killer cells and interleukin-2 or high-dose interleukin-2 alone. *New Engl J Med* 316: 889–892
17. Cortesina GA, De Stefani M, Giovarelli MG, Barioglio GP, Cavallo G, C Jemma and G Forni. Treatment of recurrent squamous cell carcinoma of head and neck with low doses of interleukin-2 (IL-2) injected perilymphatically. *Cancer* (in press)
18. Nossal GJV (1988) Triumphs and trials of immunology in the 1980s. *Immunology Today* 9: 286–291
19. Rygaard J, Povlsen CO (1969) Heterotransplantation of a human malignant tumor to 'nude' mice. *Acta Pathol Microbiol Scand* (A) 77: 758–760
20. Arione R, Jemma C, Forni M, Marchese C, Benetton G, Giubellino C, Modesti A, Martinotti MG, Cordero di Montezemolo L, Musso T and Forni G (1988) A new childhood T-cell lymphoma established in nude mice and 'in vitro'. *Cancer Res* 48: 1312–1318

The use of animals in cancer chemotherapy

T.A. CONNORS
Toxicology Unit, Medical Research Council, Carshalton, Surrey, UK

Like most drug development programmes cancer chemotherapy covers three broad areas, screening, analogue synthesis and rational drug design. The aim of large scale empirical screening is to discover 'lead' compounds which will form the basis for analogue synthesis. Analogues of the 'lead' chemical are evaluated in the hope that some will be more clinically useful because they are more selective (i.e. have fewer side effects at the effective dose) or for instance maintain their activity when given orally. Once some information has been obtained on how the drug works it may then be possible to design new types of agent which may have superior qualities (referred to as rational design).

In order to do this research, laboratory models must be available which are reliable predictors for anticancer activity in humans. In fact over the past forty years a great variety of tests have been developed as assays for anticancer agents and are summarised in Table 1. It can be seen that tests may be quite simple using cells in culture or quite complex when human tumours are transplanted to immunodeficient mice. Today about forty chemicals are useful in the treatment of cancer and when used in combination with other drugs (and often with other treatments such as surgery, radiotherapy and bone marrow transplantation) have major activity (cures or a high percentage of complete remissions) in about 14 different types of cancer (Table 2).

It is of interest to see how important animal models have been in obtaining these results and to predict in the light of past experience whether the emphasis on animal investigations rather than *in vitro* studies will increase or decrease in the future.

Although the aim of screening tests is to obtain novel structures with antitumour activity, it should be emphasised that by no means all of the present day classes of chemical were discovered as the result of empirical screening using animals. Many 'lead' compounds including the first 'lead' alkylating agent (HN2), antimetabolite (methotrexate) and platinum complex (cisplatin) were tested in tumour bearing animals because either clinical or experimental observations of some of their biological properties suggested that they should be tested for their anticancer activity. Entirely empirical testing,

S. Garattini (ed.), The Importance of Animal Experimentation for Safety and Biomedical Research, 133–140.

Table 1. Test systems have been used to 'screen' chemicals for their potential antitumour activity

A. *Miscellaneous*

Biological properties associated with anti-cancer action

1. Mutagenicity
2. Carcinogenicity
3. Prophage activation
4. Other genotoxic properties (e.g. unscheduled DNA synthesis)
5. Immunosuppressions
6. Myelosuppression
7. Foetotoxicity
8. Inhibition of glycolysis
9. Inhibition of certain enzymes (e.g. Xanthine oxidase)

B. *In vitro tests*

B1. Non tumour systems

1. Bacteriophage
2. Bacteria
3. Fungi
4. Growing root tips and stems
5. Seedlings
6. Amoeba
7. Slime moulds

B2. Tumour systems

1. Malignant cell lines (from a variety of vertebrate sources)
2. Human tumour on chorioallantoic membrane
3. Tumour cell spheroids
4. Human tumour biopsies

C. *In vivo tests*

1. Induced tumours	– chemically induced
	– induced by radiation
	– virally induced
2. Spontaneous tumours	– mammary cancer in C^{+} mice
	– leukaemia in AKR mice
3. Transplanted tumours	– Hundreds of different tumours in rat, mouse, rabbit, guinea-pig, hamster, fowl and dog

that is the very large scale screening of randomly selected chemicals, has not been very efficient selecting only a few lead chemicals, for example the nitrosoureas (BCNU), triazenes (dacarbazine) and the melamines (hexamethylmelamine). Tests using transplanted tumours have, however, been very useful in confirming activity of some classes of chemical first shown to be active *in vitro* e.g. the actinomycins and in the further analysis of the chemicals referred to above, e.g. HN2 and cisplatin. It is in fact difficult to see how any of the present day chemicals would have had clinical trials had they not

Table 2. Diseases which respond to cancer chemotherapy (a high proportion of cures or significant extension of disease-free survival time). The components of drug combinations are listed. Sometimes these are part of combined therapies (surgery and radiation treatment) and may be used with rescue agents (e.g. bone marrow transplantation after high-dose cyclophosphamide or leucovorin rescue after high-dose methotrexate.)

Cancer type	Chemical
Acute lymphocytic leukaemia	Adriamycin, asparagenase, daunorubicin, methotrexate, prednisolone, vincristine
Hodgkin's disease	Adriamycin, bleomycin, cyclophosphamide, dacarbazine, HN_2, prednisone, procarbazine, vincristine, vinblastine
Choriocarcinoma	Actinomycin D, methotrexate
Testicular cancer	Actinomycin D, bleomycin, cyclophosphamide, cisplatin, etoposide, vinblastine
Wilms' tumour	Actinomycin D, adriamycin, vincristine
Embryonal rhabdomyosarcoma	Actinomycin D, adriamycin, cyclophosphamide, vincristine
Ewing's sarcoma	Adriamycin, cyclophosphamide, vincristine
Hairy cell leukaemia	Deoxycoformycin, interferon
Non Hodgkin's lymphoma	Cyclophosphamide, cytosine, arabinoside, methotrexate, vincristine
Diffuse histocytic lymphoma	Adriamycin, bleomycin, cyclophosphamide, etoposide, HN_2, methotrexate, prednisone, procarbazine, vincristine
Osteogenic sarcoma	Actinomycin D, adriamycin, bleomycin, cisplatin, cyclophosphamide, ifosfamide, melphalan, methotrexate, mitomycin C
Acute myelocytic leukaemia	Adriamycin, cyclophosphamide, cytosine, arabinoside, thioguanine
Breast cancer	Tamoxifen, progestins, aminoglutethimide, adriamycin, cyclophosphamide, 5-fluorouracil, methotrexate, prednisone
Small cell lung cancer	Adriamycin, cyclophosphamide, cisplatin, etoposide, lomustine, methotrexate, vincristine

shown activity against tumour bearing animals. A compound selected by *in vitro* screening by virtue of its high toxicity would be unlikely to be developed clinically had it not been subsequently shown to have good antitumour activity in animals. Some useful agents such as methotrexate are not particularly potent and would not necessarily have been selected by *in vitro* systems. A particular problem of *in vitro* screening is that it is now known that some useful anticancer agents require activation by liver microsomes to generate the true anticancer metabolite. The triazenes and melamines are two examples of where clinically useful agents would have been lost by *in vitro* testing since neither of these agents (which are in effect prodrugs) are very toxic to cells in culture. The best known example is cyclophosphamide, one of the most useful of present day agents. Early members of the cyclophosphamide series designed to be selectively activated by tumour cells were tested only against cells in culture and the idea was not pursued after a number of negative results. It was only when cyclophosphamide was later tested in animals with transplanted tumours that it was realised that metabolism in the liver was an essential first stage in the activation process.

Tumour bearing animals are useful for 'ranking' analogues in order of their effectiveness. By measurement of the therapeutic index (a ratio of toxic or lethal dose to the tumour effective dose) the potentially most useful analogues of a large series can be selected. A comparable experiment *in vitro* would be to compare the tumour cell with a 'normal' cell line and while this can be attempted if the normal target cell has already been determined (from an animal toxicity experiment), two of the major advantages of *in vitro* tests, speed and cheapness, are lost if the system becomes complicated. Major advances in cancer chemotherapy have come from the use of drugs in combination and from the use of optimum dose schedules for each anticancer agent, particularly important for phase specific agents such as cytosine arabinoside where variation in dose schedule can greatly affect the antitumour activity of the drug. Because of the large number of variables involved the tumour bearing animal is the only possible model to study complicated drug combinations and dose schedules.

Both *in vivo* and *in vitro* models have been used to investigate 'rationally' synthesised drugs, the most important being targetted drugs or prodrugs which are relatively non-toxic agents which are designed to be specifically metabolised by tumour enzymes to release a toxic metabolite. *In vitro* and *in vivo* tests are used in a complementary fashion. The drug is first assayed *in vitro* against cells which are high or low in the appropriate activating enzyme, or which are highly or poorly targetted by the drug. If a good differential cell kill is obtained the prodrug is examined in animals with tumours. In this case initial testing against cells *in vitro* is appropriate, because the mechanism by which the agent acts is known.

Cancer chemotherapy and the future

Despite the central role of tumour bearing rodents in the past development of anticancer agents, future work planned in the light of results obtained over the past twenty years suggests that the use of transplanted tumour systems and other animal models will diminish considerably over the next decade.

The approach which uses by far the greatest number of animals is empirical screening. In retrospect a serious drawback of this approach has been that it has only selected chemicals which act by a common antiproliferative mechanism. Figure 1 shows the classes of chemical that have been used clinically since 1950. All of them act by interfering with precise events in nucleic acid and protein synthesis. Interference with the pathways will of course be particularly toxic for cells in cycle or poliferating cells. Agents of this type

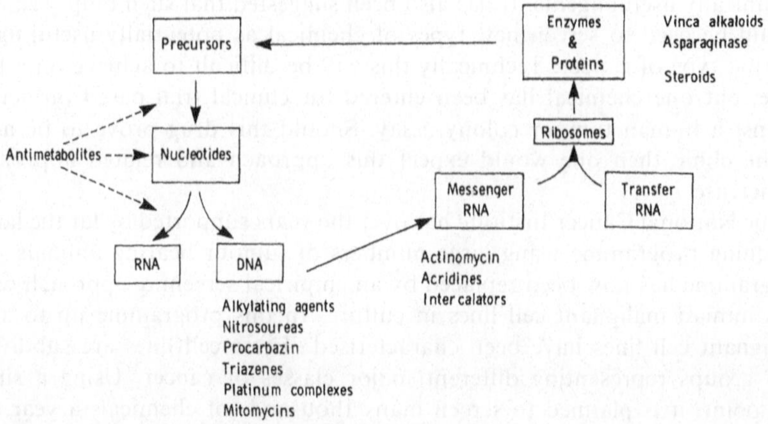

Fig. 1. Sites of action of anticancer agents.

have been used with considerable success against certain types of cancer (Table 2) but they have not been very effective against some of the most commonly occurring cancers, for example those of the lung and gastrointestinal tract. This failure to treat common cancers by chemotherapy has led to a reassessment of drug development programmes and to the investigation of alternative methods of screening for new types of agent.

The rapidly growing transplanted tumours have been the cornerstone of cell drug development programmes and it is perhaps not surprising that they have been useful in selecting only antiproliferative agents. It has been suggested that slowly growing solid tumours should be the basis for the new screening programme and while an interesting new class of anticancer agent, the flavone acetic acids, have been discovered by this approach, there is no strong evidence to suggest that future testing on mice with slowly growing transplanted tumours will provide new classes of anticancer agent.

In the human tumour xenograft system different types of human tumour are transplanted to immunodeficient mice. These slowly growing solid tumours often retain much of their original characteristics and might be the obvious replacement for animal tumours for large scale screening. However xenograft systems have been fairly intensively studied for the past fifteen years and they have not yet been responsible for discovering any new class of agent. Furthermore some chemicals which have been found to be very active against certain types of xenograft have not proved to be useful when tested in the clinic against tumours of the same histological type.

Because of the lack of animal systems obviously superior to transplanted tumours, most emphasis will probably be placed on *in vitro* systems or other methods of selection.

For some time now attempts have been made to select the best drug combinations for individual cancer patients, by removing a biopsy of the tumour prior to chemotherapy and assessing its chemosensitivity to a range of clinically useful agents. It has also been suggested that such biopsy samples should be used to screen new types of chemical as potentially useful agents for that type of cancer. Technically this will be difficult to achieve on a large scale, but one chemical has been entered for clinical trial based on activity against a human tumour colony assay. Should this drug prove to be active in the clinic then one would expect this approach and related approaches to increase.

The National Cancer Institute has over the years supported by far the largest screening programme using large numbers of tumour bearing animals. This programme has now been replaced by an empirical screening approach which uses human malignant cell lines in culture. In this programme up to a 100 malignant cell lines have been characterised. These cell lines are subdivided into groups representing different major classes of cancer. Using a simple end point, it is planned to screen many thousands of chemicals a year. The primary aim is to discover 'disease specific drugs', that is chemicals which have a selective toxicity to one of the sub-groups described above which are made up of representatives of one cancer type. This approach if successful in discovering new treatments for say lung or GI tract cancer would almost certainly become the accepted method for looking for 'lead' compounds and would greatly reduce the numbers of animals used in experimental cancer chemotherapy.

The Cancer Research Campaign (CRC) of the UK have developed a radical approach to the selection of new agents for clinical trial and is based on the view that animal models previously used in screening will not provide chemicals useful in the treatment of common solid cancers. Agents are selected for clinical trial based on the criteria of Table 3. Preferred drugs will be those of a novel chemical structure (analogues of known active chemicals will thus have only a low priority) with a unique biological action, for example activity against slowly but not rapidly growing tumours (for example flavone acetic acid) or against a spectrum of particular human xenografts or against a particular cell type. Facilities are available to synthesise selected chemicals in ample amounts and to carry out formulation, preclinical toxicology, Phase I and a limited number of Phase II clinical trials. The innovative aspect of the CRC scheme (apart from the method of selection of the useful chemicals) is that the toxicology protocols rely on one month toxicity data in mice which

Table 3. Rationale for the selection of the chemicals for clinical trial by the CRC Phase I Committee

1. Novel chemical structure. Not acting as an anti-proliferative agent.
2. Unusual antitumour activity. For example, active against slowly growing but not rapidly growing rodent transplanted tumour. Selective effect on particular classes of human tumour xenograft.
3. Selective toxicity to stem cells or a particular cell type or organ.
4. Adequate drug available or available through synthesis.
5. Clinicians interested in organising the Phase I clinical trial.

includes pharmacokinetic data together with LD_{10} determination in mice and rats. This protocol is based on the argument that there is sufficient past experience of Phase I clinical trials, much of it recorded in the literature, to suggest that extensive toxicological testing is not required in the case of Phase I clinical trials of anticancer agents. There is no need for toxicological data on mammals other than rodents and the use of dogs as recommended by some countries is unnecessary. The system has been operating successfully since the early 1980's and to date around twenty new agents are awaiting or have been used successfully in Phase I/II clinical trials.

It is also likely that fewer animals will be used to test analogues in the future. In the past many hundreds of analogues of a 'lead' chemical have been synthesised in the search for better agents. From past experience this has clearly been a wasteful process since as already mentioned the earliest members of the series (HN2, methotrexate, adriamycin, vinblastine, cisplatin) have still not been replaced by later analogues showing that the fairly random synthesis of analogues is not very productive. In the future analogue synthesis will probably proceed more rationally. Early on some idea of the target site of a lead chemical will come from basic research and this knowledge will be combined with computer graphics and modelling to predict more effective analogues. Nevertheless animals will continue to be used for the development of 'second generation' agents. Once a chemical has been extensively evaluated in the clinic its disadvantages, particularly the serious toxicity it causes to vital organs, will become well known. Attempts will then be made in the laboratory to determine whether analogues can be found which have similar antitumour action but do not cause such serious side effects. Adriamycin for example is a very useful anticancer agent but at high doses it is cardiotoxic. Analogues of adriamycin might be tested in animals with tumours to see if they maintain antitumour effectiveness but have less cardiotoxicity. *In vitro* systems which can readily give this sort of information do not exist at present. Cisplatin is an essential component of drug combinations used with great success for the treatment of testicular cancer. Being a heavy metal it not unexpectedly causes irreversible toxicity to kidney and peripheral nerves. Screening of a series of analogues against mice, looking particularly for those that caused little nephrotoxicity led to the discovery of carboplatin, an analogue which is as efficacious as cisplatin but at the maximum tolerated doses causes the more easily handled bone marrow toxicity rather than nephrotoxicity or ototoxicity.

Rational synthesis will continue to use a mixture of *in vitro* and *in vivo* tests. Drug targetting concentrates on monoclonal antibodies to human tumours, which are used to carry radioisotopes, cytotoxic agents, toxins or enzymes to the appropriate tumour. Preliminary tests compare the cytotoxicity of the targetted agent against tumour cells with and without the appropriate antigen to determine whether effective targetting occurs. An essential second stage before clinical trial would then be further studies in mice bearing the appropriate human tumours as a xenograft. Prodrug design is nowadays more directed to the treatment of human solid cancers and in one programme prodrugs are being synthesised which will be selectively activated by hypoxic cells which invariably occur in tumours once they have reached a certain size. Early tests to select the best prodrugs measure toxicity in oxic and hypoxic cells *in vitro* but before clinical trials one would need some evidence that there was selective activity by hypoxic tumour cells *in vivo* and this would require the use of tumour bearing animals.

Conclusions

Future progress in cancer chemotherapy will depend on the use of animals and particularly tumour bearing rodents. However if the *in vitro* screening systems now being developed are successful, most of the investigations using animals will be confined to relatively small-scale studies on analogues and rationally designed prodrugs or targetted drugs. The new toxicology protocols first used by the CRC and now being adopted by other organisations will also result in a reduced requirement for toxicity testing with higher mammals, such as dogs, no longer being required.

The use of experimental animals in transplantation research

D.W. VAN BEKKUM
Radiobiological Institute TNO, Rijswijk, The Netherlands

The development of transplantation biology

Research into organ and tissue transplantation has been going on for more than a century, but it did not acquire the status of a separate discipline until the early fifties when the first international meetings on this subject were organised. The first Tissue Homo transplantation conference of the New York Academy of Science took place in 1954 and the Transplantation Society was founded as an international scientific body in 1966.

The surgical technique of vascular anastomosis, designed in 1902 by Alexis Carrel, opened the way to the experimental study of the biology of organ transplantation. It took half a century of research before the first clinical kidney transplants became successful. In 1954 the teams of Hume in Boston and of Hamburger in Paris both utilised identical twin donors and obtained prolonged functional survival of renal grafts. It should be noted here that kidney transplantation only became technically feasible after the introduction of haemodialysis machines. With that device, originally termed 'artificial kidney', invented by Kolff, it became possible to keep patients with renal insufficiency alive until transplantation of a donor kidney could be performed.

By that time it had become sufficiently clear from the research of immunologists and geneticists that a graft from any other donor than one genetically identical with the recipient will be rejected. The immunological nature of this rejection required extensive studies with laboratory mice which were successfully performed by Peter Medawar and his group in the fifties. It is important to note that tens of thousands of burned patients were available for any kind of experiments aimed at improving the therapeutic effect of skin grafts and that nonetheless the problems could not be solved without a great deal of basic research involving laboratory animals.

Among laboratory rodents it is now easy to obtain such so-called syngeneic animals in large numbers since it has become the custom to produce laboratory mice and rats in a genetically pure form, that is by continuous brother and sister mating to a high degree of inbreeding. Because of this, it became feasible to study the role of genetic factors in any type of experimental set-up. The

S. Garattini (ed.), The Importance of Animal Experimentation for Safety and Biomedical Research, 141–151.

selection of genetically homogenous strains of mice and later of rats got its stimulus from the need to study genetic influence on susceptibility to cancer induction. This development was enforced by the use of inbred strains for transfer of tumours and their unique feasibility for the study of tissue transplantation. The availability of these inbred strains made it worth while to develop microsurgical techniques that allowed kidney, heart and liver transplantation in small laboratory animals thus reducing the need for dogs and monkeys.

Among humans, syngeneic individuals are extremely rare; only 1 in 270 pregnancies results in a pair of identical twins. In the majority of instances, only the organs of unrelated persons are available and these are normally rejected within 14 days after transplantation. Two methods have been employed, separately and in combination, to prevent rejection.

One approach is to treat the recipient with immunosuppressive agents, the second to select donors who share certain tissue antigens with the recipients. Tissue antigens are not only present in various cells of the organs, but also on white blood cells, just as blood group antigens are present on the surface of red blood cells. The tissue type of a person can therefore be determined in a small sample of peripheral blood. The development of techniques by which the various tissue types could be distinguished was initiated in 1954 by Dausset [1] and has developed into a sophisticated methodology of tissue typing by which the best matches between available kidneys and potential recipients can be determined. The more compatible the donor is, the less rejection problems are to be expected. The tissue antigens involved are called histocompatibility antigens or leukocyte antigens and the genes that are involved in the coding of these antigens are histocompatibility genes. However, even the best possible matching (except in the case of syngeneity) does not prevent rejection unless immunosuppressive treatment is given. The first agent with a strong immunosuppressive activity was discovered by Schwarz and Dameshek [2] in 1958 when they found that 6-mercaptopurine inhibited antibody formation. Before that, numerous attempts had been made to utilise various forms of irradiation, such as total body irradiation, partial body irradiation, or organ irradiation, in attempts to exploit its immunosuppressive effects. However, this approach did not result in a practical treatment because of either too much toxicity or not enough suppression.

Pharmacological immunosuppression became the method of choice when 6-mercaptopurine was replaced by a more effective analog, azathioprine (Imuran), and combined with corticosteroids. During the sixties there was great interest in the development of antilymphocytic sera, some of which had an excellent effect in suppressing the allograft reaction [3]. Presently, these are being replaced by monoclonal antibodies which have the advantage of greater uniformity and reproducibility. In the seventies, a powerful new immunosuppressive compound Cyclosporin A was introduced by Borel [4]. This and a number of other technical developments have improved the long term results of organ grafts to such an extent that organ grafting has become a very attractive treatment for an ever increasing number of life-threatening diseases. Presently, more than 25,000 kidneys are being grafted annually throughout the world. About 22% of patients in treatment for end-stage renal disease in Europe carry a functioning kidney transplant. The corresponding figure for the U.S.A. is not available but is probably in the same range. It seems therefore that the number of kidney transplantations will increase further in the next years, especially when the age limit for recipients is increased as it was many years ago in Scandinavia [5]. Other organs that are being increasingly transplanted now are hearts, heart and lung combinations, pancreas and liver. Several thousands of these transplantations are performed annually and as the results improve the indications for these applications are widening. Until last year more than 10,000 allogeneic bone marrow transplantations had been performed and the annual number is increasing steeply.

Table 1. Development and advances in organ transplantation that depended on research with animals

Period studies were initiated or peaked	Subject of studies	Species
pre-1900	skin grafting	sheep, dogs, rodents, humans
1900-1910	surgical anastomosis of blood vessels	dogs
1910-1940	rejection of allografts of tumours, skin and organs	many species, including chicken embryos
1940-1950	proof for immunological nature of allograft rejection, second set phenomenon, transfer of immunity, development of haemodialysis	human (skin), mice dogs, large animals
1950-1960	immunosuppression with radiation and chemical agents genetic basis of rejection leukocyte antigens development of microsurgical techniques	human subjects, dogs, mice, rats, monkeys
1960-1970	Graft-versus-Host Disease anti-lymphocytic antibodies liver, heart, pancreas transplantation, tissue typing	dogs, monkeys, horses, goats, rodents, humans
1970-present	new area of immunology Cyclosporin A, monoclonal antibodies lymphocyte depletion in bone marrow grafting, clinical application of transplantation of many organs	mice, rats, rabbits, dogs, monkeys, humans animal models of specific human diseases

For each step in the development of organ and tissue transplantation, experimentation with animals has been of vital importance. In many countries it is considered unethical to introduce a new procedure like kidney or heart transplantation in the clinic until convincing evidence has been obtained in animals that acceptable results may be expected.

In Table 1 a listing has been provided of the various animal species that were involved in the subsequent stages of research on transplantation. In the following paragraph we shall describe the research on bone marrow transplantation, to illustrate the role of experimental animals in developing this treatment into a clinically useful practice.

The use of experimental animals in bone marrow transplantation research

The line of investigation which eventually led to the discovery of bone marrow transplantation originated from the intensification of the studies on the effects of ionizing radiation on the mammalian organism in connection with the development of nuclear weapons during World War II. Many animal species, from large ones such as cows and burros to the small rodents, were exposed to high dose radiation to unravel the cause of radiation sickness and ensuing death. It was soon established that there were important differences between the species in sensitivity to whole body irradiation. The LD_{50} of animals the size of humans was lower (in the order of 3–4 Gy) than that of mice and rats (about 6–7 Gy). It also became clear that mortality was the result of a dramatic decrease in peripheral blood granulocytes, lymphocytes and platelets. The exposed animals died either from haemorrhages or from infections caused by microorganisms that normally are not pathogenic. The pancytopenia was caused by destruction of the haemopoietic tissues which are among the most radiosensitive in the body. Jacobson *et al.* [6] discovered in 1949 that shielding of one whole leg or the spleen of mice during exposure to a lethal dose of whole body irradiation caused an impressive reduction in mortality. Moreover, the spleen appeared to be specific in this respect, since shielding of other organs was not effective with the exception of shielding of a whole leg.

The choice of the experimental animal, the mouse, in these investigations was an exceptionally fortunate one, but not unusual since mice have been the most frequently employed laboratory mammals. In the mouse, the spleen is essentially a haemopoietic organ very similar to the bone marrow, while in rats, guinea pigs, rabbits and in the larger laboratory animal species the spleen is strictly a lymphatic tissue. Jacobson's results therefore emphasized the significance of the damage to the haemopoietic system for the development of that particular form of radiation sickness which is now generally known as the 'bone marrow syndrome'.

In the experiments described above, the spleen was exteriorised to permit effective and selective shielding and every attempt was made to maintain the blood supply of the spleen during this procedure. In some cases, however, the spleen was found to be completely infarcted on completion of the irradiation. It was nevertheless returned to the abdominal cavity and much to the surprise of the investigators, these animals were subsequently found to be as well protected as the mice in which the blood supply to the spleen had not been interrupted. From this, Jacobson drew the conclusion that an infarcted spleen was probably equivalent to a spleen autograft in protective capacity and this led him to study the effects of implantation of autologous and syngeneic spleens and, when these proved to be effective, of spleen fragments and cell suspensions of spleen and bone marrow.

By 1955 other laboratories had confirmed and extended these observations and it was well established that the implantation or intravenous infusion of haemopoietic cells after lethal whole body irradiation was highly effective in preventing mortality, by inducing the rapid recovery of haemopoiesis.

At that time many investigators favoured the idea that this therapeutic effect of bone marrow (and mouse spleen) cells was due to a humoral factor produced by or present in these tissues, that stimulated the few surviving haemopoietic cells of the irradiated recipient into accelerated proliferation and repopulation. This notion was based on the observation that allogeneic and even xenogeneic (rat into mouse) bone marrow infusions were also highly protective. It was considered highly unlikely that non-identical cells would survive and proliferate, since grafting of many other tissues, notably skin, had uniformly failed, except between genetically identical individuals.

It was therefore quite a break-through when in 1956 convincing evidence was provided by three different teams of investigators [7–9] that the transplanted haemopoietic cells proliferate and establish themselves in the depleted bone marrow cavities of the recipient, thereby eventually replacing the whole haemopoietic and immunological system. This discovery not only paved the way for bone marrow transplantation in patients, but also for a new and very profitable methodology that allowed cellular descendance in the immunohaemopoietic system to be traced by the use of genetic markers.

The term haemopoietic chimaera or radiation chimaera was introduced to describe the result of a successful allo- or xenograft of bone marrow cells, because one was in fact dealing with a mouse that was for the rest of its life producing foreign erythrocytes, lymphocytes, platelets and many other donor derived cells, and survived by virtue of this continuing production.

Radiation chimaeras have become invaluable for unravelling the cellular hierarchy of the haemopoietic system and for the study of immune functions. One of the most important subsequent discoveries was the observation of colonies of cells in the form of macroscopic nodules in the spleen about 10 days after a mouse has been irradiated and given an intravenous graft of a small number of bone marrow cells. These nodules harbour a colony of cells and are of many haemopoietic differentiation lines, all derived from a single precursor cell [10].

Moreover, it was shown that the cells of a single spleen nodule can repopulate and cure a lethally irradiated syngeneic mouse recipient [11]. This finding demonstrated that a single primitive precursor cell can generate a complete haemopoietic/lymphatic system consisting of 10^9 cells (in the mouse) of all differentiation types. This mother cell or pluripotent stem cell (PHSC) constitutes an extremely low percentage (less than 1%) of the bone marrow. Much effort was directed toward concentration, purification and eventual identification by morphological characterizations or cell surface markers of the PHSC [12]. The most rapid progress could be made in mice and rats because in other species the functional tests for PHSC i.e. spleen colony assays and capacity for radiation protection are either not operational or far too labourious and expensive. If laboratory mice and rats had not been available for this type of research, our present-day haematology would have remained at the level of 1950. The information that is most sought after is on the identity, the frequency and other characteristics of the human PHSC, as well as on the regulation of stem cell replication and differentiation in health and disease. Most of this information has to be derived from rodent data but the translation to human haemopoiesis has been greatly facilitated by the introduction of methods for the *in vitro* culture of bone marrow cells which allow the identification of a variety of restricted clonogenic stem cells [13].

Just this year McCune *et al.* [14] reported the take and proliferation of human haemopoietic stem cells in non-irradiated mice of a very special strain called SCID, that has hereditary immunodeficiency for both the T and B cell functions. Perhaps with this mouse assay system it will be feasible to enumerate human PHSC by *in vivo* functional end points.

All the progress described above has depended heavily on severely immunosuppressed mice. It soon became clear that supralethally irradiated mice – needed for spleen colony assays and repopulation studies – are extremely vulnerable to infections. These infections are caused by microorganisms already present in the host or its microenvironment e.g. the gut or the skin or by microorganisms from outside, to which immunocompetent individuals are normally resistant. The need to prevent such infections from interfering with the results of the studies led to the introduction of specific pathogen-free mice and rats in research institutions engaged in radiation research, immunology, experimental haematology and transplantation biology. The elimination of the normal pathogens proved to be not enough. Even pathogen-free animals could die early after irradiation from infection with *Enterobacteriaceae* normally present in the gut. Attempts were therefore made to produce laboratory animals with a restricted gut flora, excluding all bacterial species that caused complications after heavy immunosuppressive treatment. Needless to say, this development has greatly influenced the level of sophistication and thereby the efforts and costs involved in producing these animals. It also follows that a high priority is given to any method that can replace PHSC assays in living mice [15].

The further development of clinical bone marrow transplantation

Once it had been established that production of haemopoietic chimaeras is feasible, the many desirable clinical applications of this principle were immediately recognized. In essence, many if not all diseases originating in the haemopoietic tissue would become curable by replacing the diseased cells with PHSC derived from a healthy donor, i.e. aplastic anaemia, leukaemia and many hereditary diseases of haemopoiesis or the immune system. However, there were a number of serious obstacles to be removed before this dream could come true. Soon after the discovery of chimerism, it became apparent that a major complication occurred in many instances of initially successful grafts of allo- (and xeno)geneic bone marrow. The grafted mice first fully reconstituted their bone marrow and then developed a disease characterized by lesions in the skin (dermatitis), the gut (diarrhoea) and the liver (hepatitis). This disease could follow an acute or a chronic course and carried a high risk of mortality. It was shown to be caused by donor-type lymphocytes that were able to mount an immunological reaction against the tissues of the recipient and the disease was called Graft-versus-Host Disease (GvHD). For more detailed reviews on GvHD the reader is referred to [16, 17].

The first attempts at transplantation of mismatched bone marrow in the treatment of leukaemia did not result in any long term survival because of this complication. Following the introduction of techniques for matching with human leukocyte antigens (HLA), so-called HLA identical sibling donors were used and this gave better results. Nonetheless, severe GvHD occurred in 50% of these cases and half of the patients with GvHD died from this complication. While GvHD in mice had a delayed and chronic pattern, GvHD in human patients was usually of an acute and severe character. Obviously, there existed important differences between mouse and man, and to conquer the problems arising from GvHD in man, an animal model that would react more like humans had to be introduced.

After comparing human haematology and immunology with that of the two classical candidate species for preclinical studies, the rhesus monkey and the dog, we chose to concentrate on monkeys, mostly because the existing body of knowledge on that species was greater than that on dogs. Our group began experimental bone marrow transplantation in the rhesus monkey at the end of the fifties. At the same time Thomas and Ferrebee in the U.S.A. started similar research in dogs. In both species, tissue typing methodology was developed along the same lines as in humans. The dog model had the advantages that large groups of siblings can be bred relatively easily because of its large litter size and that dogs mature faster than monkeys. The need for MHC identical sibling donor recipient combinations required breeding colonies of both dogs and monkeys.

For the latter species there were additional compelling reasons for setting up laboratory breeding. Firstly, the availability of monkeys captured in the wild was declining rapidly and several exporting countries were already limiting their supplies. Secondly, the captured monkeys harboured a variety of infectious diseases such as shigella, salmonellae and tuberculosis as well as several persistent intestinal parasites. Among the latter Oesophagostomum apiostomum which causes inflammatory nodules in the wall of the intestines proved to be a frequent source of bacterial complications (peritonitis and septic anaemia) following high-dose irradiation. Laboratory bred monkeys can be kept free of such infections and parasites. The large scale laboratory breeding of subhuman primates that has become common practice in some Western countries has improved the quality of the animals, reduced the number of animals needed for the experiments and has nearly abolished the demand for importing animals captured in the wild.

Within a few years after the identification of GvHD as an immunological reaction of the grafted cells or their descendants against the recipient [18], we established in the mouse model that the incidence and severity of the GvHD are directly related to the number of lymphoid cells grafted with the bone marrow [19]. These experiments were performed by adding lymph node cells or spleen cells to the bone marrow graft. When a sufficiently large number of lymphoid cells were added, the recipients developed the same severe and acute type of GvHD as was seen in human patients grafted with mismatched allogeneic bone marrow. Because of this severe complication and its ensuing high mortality, clinical bone marrow transplantation was for many years restricted to MHC-identical sibling recipient-donor combinations. The patients were also routinely treated with the immunosuppressive drug methotrexate, which resulted in an incidence of GvHD of 50% and a mortality related to GvHD of 25%. In the large animal models the influence of MHC matching could be studied without added immunosuppressive treatment. Under these conditions the incidence of severe fatal GvHD in rhesus monkeys is 90%. In dogs transplantation of MHC-matched sibling marrow results in about 50% GvHD, its severity is less and the disease is usually not fatal. In MHC-identical mouse combinations GvHD does not usually complicate bone marrow transplantation. The different responses of these species can be fully explained by taking into account the differences in the proportion of T-lymphocytes in their bone marrow. Primates have up to 30% T-lymphocytes in their bone marrow, rodents only 1–2% and the bone marrow of dogs contains an intermediate proportion.

The logical consequence of these observations on the crucial role of T-lymphocytes as the cause of GvHD is that GvHD should be prevented by removal or inactivation of these cells from the bone marrow graft prior to transplantation. In 1968 we developed a method [20] which permitted the separation of lymphocytes responsible for inducing GvHD from the cells required to repopulate the immunohaemopoietic system of lethally irradiated mice. Subsequently, this method was adapted to the bone marrow of monkeys, dogs and humans and it became fully established that T-lymphocyte depletion is highly effective in preventing GvHD. In recent years inactivation of T-lymphocytes with monoclonal antibodies alone or in combination with physical methods of separation is being employed. The monkey model has been very useful in predicting the degree of depletion required to prevent GvHD in matched as well as in mismatched combinations in human patients.

In the course of the experiments with T cell depleted bone marrow grafts in monkeys and dogs, we noticed an increased proportion of graft failures compared to transplantation of unmodified bone marrow. This was in a sense to be expected since the GvHD reaction is also directed against the surviving T-lymphocytes of the recipient and adds to the general immunosuppression of the recipient. We were able to demonstrate that this problem can be overcome by increasing the dose of total body irradiation (TBI) by about 2 Gy. In order to avoid toxicity of this higher dose of TBI, it was shown in both dogs and monkeys that TBI should be given in two fractions separated by 24 h. or 72 h. [21, 22]. Many clinical teams have introduced T cell depletion in their bone marrow transplantation protocol and when properly applied have reported a virtual absence of GvHD in MHC-matched sibling combinations [23, 24]. However, those transplant teams who have not adapted their conditioning regimen so as to provide additional immunosuppression have encountered an unacceptable incidence of graft failures. These teams are also reporting an increased incidence of leukaemia relapses when using T cell depleted marrow grafts in the treatment of leukaemia. It has been known for some time that the relapse rate is much lower among bone marrow transplantation patients who have suffered from GvHD than among those who have not experienced GvHD. Apparently, the immune reaction against host tissues is capable of inactivating a certain number of residual leukaemia cells as well. The availability of extensive kinetic data on leukaemic regrowth after remission induction in a rat model of acute myeloid leukaemia enabled us to calculate the anti-leukaemic effect of GvHD in terms of log leukaemic cell kill [25]. It turned out that this amounts to about 1 log cell kill which is provided by the extra conditioning with a dose of 2 Gy that was recommended to avoid rejection of T cell depleted marrow.

Such important information can be derived from well designed animal models. It has served to avoid the unnecessary deterioration of clinical results that would occur if clinicians were to abandon the highly successful methods of prevention of GvHD by T cell depletion, out of concern for an increased relapse rate. It would be very difficult, requiring clinical trials with hundreds of patients, to establish the necessary modifications in the treatment protocol without the use of data from animal models. In fact, the present restrictions on the use of monkeys and dogs imposed by legal, economic and public opinion pressures, is already adversely influencing the performance of a sufficiently large number of preclinical experiments. This trend is leading to a substantial increase in avoidable human suffering and mortality.

Ongoing experimental research is directed at the safe and effective application of mismatched bone marrow grafts and at the design of less toxic regimens of conditioning of the recipients.

In addition, a new line of research has recently been developed to explore the application of bone marrow transplantation in the treatment of a group of genetically determined metabolic diseases caused by a specific lysosomal enzyme deficiency or lysosomal storage diseases. The clinical pathology of these very serious diseases is due to the absence of a single enzyme. Attempts to treat these patients with the administration of enzyme preparations have generally not yielded satisfactory results. The underlying principle of bone marrow transplantation is limited to deficiencies of those enzymes that are produced by haemopoietic cells. The successful introduction of normal bone marrow would supply the patient with a continuous source of the lacking enzyme. Many of these diseases affect the central nervous system, because toxic storage products, normally degraded by the enzyme in question, accumulate in the brain. For several of these human diseases, similar deficiencies have been discovered in animals. These provide unique models in which the pathology and its treatment can be studied without the many restrictions encountered in patients. One outstanding advantage of the animal models is that the number of animals available always greatly exceeds the number of patients, because these diseases are very rare. One important question to be answered was whether cells of the grafted bone marrow would enter the central nervous system so that the enzyme could reach this very sensitive organ. With the use of Twitcher mice, a model for galactosyl ceraminase deficiency (Krabbe's disease) in humans, it could be demonstrated that donor-derived macrophages do indeed penetrate the brain causing degradation of the toxic storage product [26].

A different approach to treatment of enzyme deficiency disease is the normalisation of the patient's cells by introducing the appropriate gene: so-called somatic gene therapy. This approach has not yet resulted in practical applications, but the bone marrow is again a very attractive target tissue for this treatment because its cellular products are distributed throughout the whole organism.

Conclusions

The need for studying prolonged states of immunosuppression has stimulated the development of specific pathogen-free animal rodent colonies and rodents with a restricted microflora. The availability of these animals has widened the possibilities for preclinical studies and greatly improved the results of organ and bone marrow transplantation. The need for clean monkeys and dogs with a known genetic constitution, mostly of MHC groups, has led to replacement of captured or collected animals by laboratory bred animals. In the case of monkeys this development has contributed to the preservation of monkeys in their native habitats.

References

1. Dausset J (1954) *Vox Sang* 4: 190
2. Schwarz R, Stark J, Dameshek W (1958) *Proc Soc Exp Biol Med* 99: 164
3. Antilymphocytic serum (1967) CIBA Found. Study Group 29, GEW Wolstenholm and M O'Connor (Eds), JA Churchill Ltd, London
4. Borel JF *et al.* (1976) *Agents Actions* 6: 648
5. Lundgren G (1987) *Transpl Proc* 14:1, 63–66
6. Jacobson LO *et al.* (1949) *Proc Soc Exp Biol Med* 70: 740–742
7. Ford *et al.* (1956) *Nature* 177: 450–454
8. Vos *et al.* (1956) *Acta Physiol Pharmacol Neerl* 4: 482–486
9. Nowell *et al.* (1956) *Cancer Res* 16: 258–261
10. Till JE and McCullouch EA (1961) *Radiation Res* 14: 213
11. Trentin JJ and Fallberg WJ (1963) In: *Conceptional Advances in Immunology and Oncology*, Texas, Harper and Row, New York
12. Van Bekkum DW, Van Noord MJ, Maat B, Dicke KA (1971) *Blood* 38: 547
13. Bradley TR and Metcalf D (1966) *J Exp Biol* 44: 287
14. McCune JM *et al.* (1988) *Science* 241: 1632
15. De Vries P (1988) Thesis, Erasmus University, Rotterdam
16. Van Bekkum DW and De Vries MJ (1967) Radiation Chimaeras, Logos Press, Academic Press
17. Van Bekkum DW (1985) Graft versus Host Disease, chapter 3. In: DW van Bekkum and B Löwenberg (Eds) *Bone Marrow Transplantation*, Marcel Dekker Inc., New York
18. Van Bekkum DW and Vos O (1957) *J Cell C Physiol* 50: 139
19. Van Bekkum DW (1964) *Transplantation* 2: 293
20. Dicke KA *et al.* (1968) *Transplantation* 6: 562
21. Wagemaker G *et al.* (1982) In: JS Baum *et al.* (Eds) *Experimental Haematology Today*, S Karger, Basel, 111
22. Walma EP *et al.* (1987) *Transplantation* 43: 818–823
23. Hagenbeek A, Löwenberg B (1987) In: Bone Marrow Transplantation 2, suppl 1, Proc of the XIIIth Annual Meeting of European Cooperative Group for BMT, 1–5 March, Interlaken, 141
24. Burnett AK *et al.* (1988) *Leukemia* 2: 300
25. Schultz FW, Vriesendorp HM, Hagenbeek A (1988) *Blood*, submitted
26. Hoogerbrugge PM (1988) Thesis, State University Leiden

Animal models for AIDS research

PETER BENTVELZEN
Radiobiological Institute TNO, Rijswijk, The Netherlands

Introduction

With the rapid increase of AIDS cases in the United States and in Europe, and the recognition of high-risk groups other than active male homosexuals, it was realized in 1982 that an infectious agent could cause the disease. Several microbial factors, including retroviruses, were suspected to be the causative agent. In order to identify the AIDS-causing agent several different animal species, including chimpanzees, were inoculated with materials such as blood from AIDS patients. These animal experiments have not yielded any worthwhile result.

One year after the recognition of the AIDS epidemic, the laboratory of L. Montagnier (Institut Pasteur, Paris) succeeded in isolating a retrovirus from peripheral blood lymphocytes of a patient with lymphadenopathy [1]. This successful isolation was the result of long-term culturing of these lymphocytes. The virus proved to be a novel retrovirus, which showed some relationship to the equine infectious anaemia virus but not to the human T cell leukaemia viruses. In 1983, Montagnier's group isolated several more of such retroviruses from AIDS patients. However, the impressive output by Gallo's laboratory (National Cancer Institute, Bethesda, Maryland) [2] has led to the rapid acceptance by the scientific community of this retrovirus, nowadays called Human Immunodeficiency Virus (HIV), as being the causative agent of AIDS.

Thanks to recombinant DNA technology the virus has been analyzed in great detail. The genomes of several HIV-isolates have been completely sequenced and there is considerable insight into the function of various HIV genes and of regulatory elements.

In order to fulfill Koch's postulates several animal species have been inoculated with an HIV-isolate. Rabbits can be infected with HIV [3]. Of the nonhuman primates only chimpanzees and gibbon apes could be infected with HIV in such a way that the virus could be reisolated from the inoculated animals [4] and that antibodies were produced against HIV proteins. However, as yet no severe morbidity has been noted in chimpanzees after an incubation period of 4–6 years. Although seroepidemiological data indicate that in man

S. Garattini (ed.), The Importance of Animal Experimentation for Safety and Biomedical Research, 153–161.

the mean incubation period for AIDS to appear is more than 6 years, it seems warranted to state that chimpanzees are relatively resistant to the pathogenic action of HIV. It would be interesting to find out why.

Although Koch's postulates were not fulfilled by means of animal experimentation, the epidemiological studies on patients who have undergone blood transfusions provide sufficient proof for the aetiological role of HIV in AIDS. The discovery of infection of rabbits with HIV came after the general acceptance by the scientific community that HIV is the causative agent of AIDS. Although animal experiments have not contributed to the discovery of HIV nor to the solution of the AIDS problem, there is a great need for animal models for some burning questions in AIDS research. Animal models are needed for the *in vivo* evaluation of antiretroviral drugs prior to clinical testing and for efficacy testing of vaccines. In addition some important questions with regard to pathogenesis remain to be solved.

Problems to be studied in animal models

What is the cause of T helper cell depletion in AIDS patients?

The severe immunodeficiency in AIDS patients is thought to be due to the severe loss of T helper lymphocytes, characterized by the CD4 cell surface molecule. *In vitro* HIV often has a strong cytopathic effect on T cell lines, which carry the CD4 cell surface antigen [5]. This finding suggests that HIV exerts its pathogenic effect *in vivo* by killing infected T helper cells. Since only a few lymphocytes of infected people contain HIV [6], the question rises how this virus could exert its pathogenic action *in vivo*. It has been suggested that HIV, which also infects cell types other than T helper cells, could affect the physiology of, for instance, follicular dendritic cells [7]. This might lead to a considerably lower production of T helper cells.

Lanzavecchia *et al.* [8] postulated that the viral envelope glycoprotein would bind to the CD4 molecule of many uninfected T helper cells. Such cells coated with viral antigen would then serve as targets for HIV-directed cytotoxic T cells.

Only experimental manipulation of infected subjects will lead to an answer to this question. This cannot be done with human beings. An appropriate animal model is needed to study this problem.

What is the cause of presenile dementia in HIV-infected individuals?

Prior to opportunistic infections behavioural changes are noted in HIV-infected individuals, in particular signs of dementia. Oedema of HIV-infected monocytic cells is found in the brain of AIDS patients [9]. Is this oedema the underlying cause of dementia?

A surprising finding was that a large part of the brain contains an antigen related to the CD4 molecule, also characteristic of T helper lymphocytes [10].

The brain-associated CD4-like molecules may also be coated with the HIV envelope glycoprotein gp120. This binding might interfere with signal transmission in the brain.

Intensive neurophysiological studies, which require invasive techniques, might give an answer to this problem. They cannot be performed on human beings and therefore an appropriate animal model is needed. In such a model not only is infection with HIV or a related virus required, but behavioural changes must also be detectable. Behavioural disturbances indicative of dementia might be observed in rodents and lagomorphs, but nonhuman primates are preferable in view of their resemblance to man.

Do microbial factors have an influence on the development of AIDS?

It has been hypothesized that prior venereal infections might facilitate the entry of HIV after sexual intercourse [11]. Various infections, such as often occur in high-risk groups like active male homosexuals or drug-addicts, might enhance the spread of HIV in an infected individual and in this way precipitate the immunodeficiency. Elegant molecular biological experiments have demonstrated that transactivating proteins from unrelated agents such as Herpes viruses may induce the expression of the HIV provirus [12]. It seems almost impossible, however, to find proof of the role of microbial factors in the development of AIDS by means of epidemiological studies. The demonstration of the role of the microflora in the precipitation of AIDS would be of great importance in the management of HIV-seropositive people. Evidently such studies must first be carried out in an animal model. As far as control of the bacterial flora is concerned the laboratory mouse constitutes the most suitable material. However, macaque species can be manipulated bacteriologically to a large extent. If one wants to study the influence of viral infections on the outcome of AIDS, nonhuman primates are the animals of choice. They usually carry viruses which are related to human viruses, such as Epstein-Barr virus and cytomegalovirus, but hand-reared monkeys lack such viruses.

Prerequisites for an animal for AIDS research

In outlining the prerequisites for an animal model for a virus disease we could not rigidly adhere to the postulates of Koch or his doctrinary followers. We have attempted, however, to follow them as closely as possible.

Productive infection is needed

A virus may infect a cell, deposit its genetic material into that of the infected cell and have its reproductive cycle blocked. Nevertheless, this nonproductive infection may have a dramatic effect like the induction of tumours in rodents by human adenoviruses or avian retroviruses. Although it has not been convincingly demonstrated, it is a reasonable assumption that only a productive infection with HIV leads to disease.

HIV can replicate *in vitro* in lymphocytes of various animal species [13] but upon inoculation it produces a productive infection in only chimpanzees, gibbon apes and rabbits. In our experience, HIV can replicate in peripheral blood lymphocytes of rhesus monkeys, but inoculation of HIV into these animals does not lead to seroconversion or to reisolation of the virus. For infection of rabbits extensive manipulation of the haemopoietic systems seems to be necessary. However, HIV seems to cause disease only in rabbits (Varnier, personal communication). With regard to Koch's postulates, the rabbit seems to be the most suitable animal for AIDS research.

The virus to be used must be HIV or as closely related to HIV as possible

Several retroviruses cause immunodeficiencies [14], although it remains to be established whether they all lead to depletion of T helper cells. In the early phases of AIDS research propaganda was made for the feline leukaemia virus which could cause serious morbidity due to opportunistic infections several years after natural infection. In the same way, type D retroviruses, which were associated with outbreaks of immunodeficiency in rhesus monkey colonies [15], have been advocated as an appropriate model for AIDS research.

Particularly for *in vivo* testing of anti-retroviral drugs, murine leukaemia viruses provide a very good model in which effects can be determined within a month. A shortcoming is that the target of most of these drugs, the viral RNA-dependent DNA polymerase (reverse transcriptase) of the murine viruses displays a different cation dependence from the HIV enzyme.

The mouse mammary tumour virus system provides worthwhile information about transmission of the virus via semen, blood and milk [16], to be used for understanding transmission of HIV. However, it would be preferable to use viruses belonging to the retrovirus genus Lentivirus as a model for HIV. The Visna/Maedi sheep virus group has provided information about antigenic variation and the role of macrophages in the spread of virus. The equine infectious anaemia virus and the caprine encephalitis arthritis virus are also of some interest to the HIV-virologist, but have little bearing upon the problem of immunodeficiency.

A lentivirus has been isolated from a cow whose immune system was impaired [17], but it still remains to be established whether this virus plays an aetiological role in immunodeficiency. No large-scale studies are presently being carried out on this so-called bovine immunodeficiency virus.

A lentivirus has also been recovered from diseased cats [18]. Seroepidemiological studies strongly indicate this virus to be an aetiological agent of immunodeficiency in cats. A pathogenic strain of this virus has not yet been isolated. Interesting studies can be performed with this feline immunodeficiency virus (FIV), taking viraemia as a biological endpoint, for instance for the testing of FIV-vaccines or of antilentivirus drugs. It would be a great advantage, however, if a pathogenic FIV strain could be isolated which could be passaged in tissue culture without losing its pathogenicity.

A retrovirus which causes immunodeficiency in rhesus monkeys has been isolated from diseased macaques [19] and from healthy sooty mangabey monkeys [20–22]. The disease does not comprise only opportunistic infections but lymphomas as well. These simian immunodeficiency viruses (SIV) are approximately 50% homologous at the nucleotide sequence level with HIV-1 and approximately 75% with HIV-2. SIV strains have been isolated from several other African monkey species but their pathogenicity in rhesus monkeys remains to be established. Most SIV strains take several months to cause disease, but one strain induces fatal disease within two weeks while another takes more than a year. Most primate centers study the SIV model in order to gain insight into the natural course of the disease, and also in order to exploit it in the near future for antiretroviral drug testing and for the development of vaccination technology.

The animal species to be used must be related to man, must be cheap and its use may not lead to its extinction

All the animal species mentioned above are mammals and in this way related to man. Obviously, the nonhuman primates, particularly the chimpanzee, are much more closely related to man than the other mammalian species such as the cat. However, the use of the chimpanzee is quite expensive. The supply of these apes for AIDS research is quite limited. Extensive use would certainly lead to its extinction. The European Community keeps 20 chimpanzees available for AIDS research at the TNO Primate Center in the Netherlands. Only a few well-chosen experiments will be carried out with these animals. Attention will be paid to providing these apes with living conditions as 'humane' as possible.

A small amount of virus can infect a chimpanzee (L.O. Arthur, personal communication). I have calculated that as little as 10^5 HIV particles would suffice and that a single infected lymphocyte may establish an infection. Chimpanzees readily seroconvert and virus can soon be reisolated from infected apes. Later on the number of virus-producing cells gradually decreases [4] and after one year HIV can only seldomly be retrieved from chimpanzees.

Unfortunately, all passive and active immunization experiments have failed to provide protection against a subsequent challenge with a small dose of HIV [23]. One reason for these frustrating failures may be that low doses of immunogen have been used. Another more likely explanation is that an HIV-variant, which is antigenically quite distinct, escapes the neutralizing antibody activity induced by the immunodominant HIV-strain. The various HIV-isolates have proved to be mixtures of quite distinct HIV-strains [24, 25].

The two macaque species which will be extensively used for AIDS research, i.e. *M. mulatta* (rhesus monkeys) and *M. fascicularis* (cynomolgus monkeys) are not endangered monkey species. They are also considerably less expensive than chimpanzees. Since SIV-infected macaques must be lodged in special biohazard-proof facilities, few animals can be used for AIDS research in a primate center. In Europe only a few hundred monkeys can therefore be infected per year with SIV or HIV-2.

Another advantage of rhesus monkeys is that like chimpanzees they share many cell surface antigens on haemopoietic cells with man. For instance, many monoclonal antibodies, which react with the CD4 marker on human T helper cells, also bind to CD4 molecules on rhesus cells.

From an economic point of view it is attractive to study AIDS in small mammals. The animals of choice would be rats and mice, because they are genetically well-defined and reagents are available to discern the various haemopoietic cell subpopulations. My laboratory is therefore engaged in attempting to adapt HIV to rodents by means of genetic manipulation. Another approach is the production of transgenic mice, which carry the HIV provirus in their germ line. Such mice are highly interesting with regard to pathogenesis, but do not provide such a realistic model. Spread of virus is not a prerequisite for the development of an immunodeficiency in such mice. Drugs interfering with 'reverse transcriptase' will not work in such mice and vaccination against HIV does not seem possible in these transgenic mice.

Rabbits can be infected with HIV but unfortunately relatively little is known about the genetics of the rabbit and no reagents are available to distinguish the various lymphocyte subpopulations.

Some strategic considerations about the use of animals for AIDS research

As mentioned above animal models are needed for solving some questions concerning the pathogenesis of AIDS, for *in vivo* evaluation of antiretroviral drugs and development of a vaccination strategy against HIV. On the basis of our present knowledge I make some recommendations as presented below.

Pathogenesis

It is recommended that HIV-infected rabbits be used whenever possible. A drawback is that despite the rabbit being the immunological workhorse for so many years, so little is known about the organization of its immune system. It remains doubtful whether the role of cytotoxic T cells directed against the HIV-glycoprotein gp120 can be determined in the rabbit. In that case one must resort to the SIV-model in macaques. It is also doubtful whether the role of other viral infections can be elucidated by using rabbits. Here again, the SIV model seems to be the best animal model.

Although many HIV-infected chimpanzees are lodged in the various primate centers, it is unlikely that these apes will be subjected to various aggressive treatments to evoke the development of AIDS. I do not know of a good hypothesis on the basis of which these apes could be subjected to a harsh regimen with the aim of inducing immunodeficiency.

Antiretroviral drugs

Drugs will first be screened *in vitro* for activity against HIV. An evaluation *in vivo* of antiretroviral activity versus toxic effects on the haemopoietic system can first be done in rodents infected with an oncovirus. However, in view of the complicated biology of lentiviruses, these drugs must be tested thereafter in HIV-infected rabbits and FIV-infected cats and finally in SIV-infected macaques. The latter also with the aim of studying toxic effects of systems other than the haemopoietic organs.

Antiviral effects might be monitored by an effect on viraemia, as presently determined by painstaking cocultivation but in the near future by a rapid molecular biological technique, the polymerase chain reaction. It is of some importance to estimate the effect on disease too. Therefore, it is necessary that reproducible immunodeficiency can be induced with a biologically defined lentivirus in either rabbits, cats or monkeys. There does not seem to be any use for chimpanzees.

The same strategy holds for various biological response modifiers, but some of the interferons can only act in a limited number of mammalian species. Human interferons may be tested in SIV-infected rhesus monkeys.

Vaccination technology

In view of the disappointing results obtained with HIV-vaccines in chimpanzees, intensive rethinking of vaccination concepts is necessary. Vaccines are needed which will provide protection against many types of HIV-1 and possibly also of HIV-2. Protection must not only be directed against virions, but also to cell-borne HIV.

Immunogenicity testing of HIV-vaccines will be done in various mammalian species, including man. The testing of HIV protein preparations in man is being carried out in several trials. The ethical value of this is questionable.

Efficacy testing can nowadays be done in rabbits. This will include testing whether a given vaccine provides protection against not only one HIV-serotype but many other HIV-strains and HIV-infected cells.

The principles involved in the preparation of a vaccine that is successful in rabbits can then be tested in the SIV-model in macaques. In my opinion, it will be unavoidable that clinical testing of an HIV vaccine is preceded by vaccination of a few chimpanzees which are subsequently challenged with a low dose of HIV. Whether or not vaccination is successful, infection with HIV does not seem to be so harmful to chimpanzees, provided they can continue to live under 'humane' conditions.

References

1. Barré-Sinoussi F, Chermann J-C, Rey F, Nugeyere MT, Chamaret S, Gruest J, Dauguet C, Axler-Blin C, Vezinet-Brun F, Rouzioux C, Rosenbaum W, Montagnier L (1983) Isolation of a lymphotropic retrovirus from a patient at risk for acquired immune deficiency syndrome (AIDS). *Science* 220: 868–871
2. Gallo RC, Salahuddin SZ, Popovic M, Shearer GM, Kaplan M, Haynes BF, Palker TJ, Redfield R, Oleske J, Safai B, White G, Foster P, Markham PD (1984) Frequent detection and isolation of cytopathic retroviruses (HTLV-III) from patients with AIDS and at risk for AIDS. *Science* 224: 500–503
3. Filice G, Cereda PM, Varnier OE (1988) Infection of rabbits with human immunodeficiency virus. *Nature* 335: 366–369
4. Fultz PN, McClure HM, Swenson RB, McGrath CR, Brodie A, Getchell JP, Jensen FC, Anderson DC, Broderson JR, Francis DP (1986) Persistent infection of chimpanzees with human T-lymphotropic virus type III/lymphadenopathy-associated virus: a potential model for acquired immunodeficiency syndrome. *J Virol* 58: 116–124
5. Lifson JD, Reyers GR, McGrath MS, Stein BS, Engleman EG (1986) AIDS retrovirus induced cytopathology: giant cell formation and involvement of the CD4 antigen. *Science* 232: 1123–1127
6. Shaw BM, Hahn BH, Arya SK, Groopman JE, Gallo RC, Wong-Staal F (1984) Molecular characterization of human T-cell leukemia (lymphotropic) virus type III in the acquired immunodeficiency syndrome. *Science* 226: 1165–1171
7. Eales L-J, Farrant J, Helbert M, Pinching AJ (1988) Peripheral blood dendritic cells in persons with AIDS and AIDS related complex: loss of high intensity class II antigen expression and function. *Clin Exp Immunol* 71: 423–427
8. Lanzavecchia A, Roosnek E, Gregory T, Berman P, Abrignani S (1988) T cells can present antigens such as HIV gp120 targeted to their own surface molecules. *Nature* 334: 530–532
9. Koenig S, Gendelman HE, Orenstein JM (1986) Detection of AIDS virus in macrophages in brain tissue from AIDS patients with encephalopathy. *Science* 233: 1089–1093
10. Maddon PJ, Dalgleish AG, McDougal JS, Clapham PR, Weiss RA, Axel R (1986) The T4 gene encodes the AIDS virus receptor and is expressed in the immune system and the brain. *Cell* 47: 333–348
11. Greenblatt RM, Lukehart SA, Plummer FA, Quinn TC, Critchlow CW, Ashley RL, D'Costa LJ, Ndinya-Achola JO, Corey L, Ronald AR, Holmes KH (1988) Genital ulceration as a risk factor for human immunodeficiency virus infection. *AIDS* 2 : 47–50
12. Ostrove JM, Leonard J, Weck KE, Rabson AB, Gendelman HE (1987) Activation of the human immunodeficiency virus by Herpes simplex virus type 1. *J Virol* 61: 3726–3732
13. McClure MD, Sattentau QJ, Beverly PCL, Hearn JP, Fitzgerald AK, Zuckerman AJ, Weiss RA (1987) HIV infection of primate lymphocytes and conservation of the CD4 receptor. *Nature* 380: 487–489
14. Bentvelzen P (1974) Comparative biology of murine and avian tumor viruses. In: Kurstak E, Maramoroschm K (eds). *Viruses, Evolution and Cancer*. Academic Press, New York pp 280–367
15. Marx PA, Maul DH, Osborn KS, Lerche NW, Moody P, Lowenstine LJ, Henrickson RV, Arthur LO, Gravell M, London WF, Sever JL, Levy JA, Munn RJ, Gardner MB (1984) Simian AIDS: isolation of a type D retrovirus and disease transmission. *Science* 223: 1083–1086
16. Bentvelzen P, Hilgers J (1980) The murine mammary tumor virus. In: Klein G (ed). *Viral Oncology*. Raven Press, New York pp 311–356
17. Van der Maaten MJ, Boothe AD, Seger CL (1972) Isolation of a virus from cattle with persistent lymphocytosis. *J Natl Cancer Inst* 49: 1649–1657
18. Pedersen N, Ho E, Brown M, Yamamoto J (1987) Isolation of a T-lymphotropic virus from domestic cats with an immunodeficiency-like syndrome. *Science* 235: 790–793

19. Daniel MD, Letvin NL, King NW, Kannagi M, Sehgal PK, Hunt RD, Kanki PJ, Essex M, Desrosiers RC (1985) Isolation of T-cell tropic HTLV-III-like retrovirus from macaques. *Science* 228: 1201–1204
20. Murphey-Corb M, Martin LN, Rangan SRS, Baskin GB, Gormus BJ, Wolf RH, Andes WA, West M, Montelaro RC (1986) Isolation of an HTLV-III related retrovirus from macaques with simian AIDS and its possible origin in asymptomatic mangabeys. *Nature* 321: 435–437
21. Fultz PN, McClure HM, Anderson DC, Swenson RB, Anand R, Srinivasan A (1986) Isolation of a T-lymphotropic retrovirus from naturally infected sooty mangabey monkeys (*Cercocebus atys*). *Proc Natl Acad Sci* USA 83: 5286–5290
22. Lowenstine LN, Pedersen NC, Higgins J, Pallis KC, Uyeda A, Marx P, Lerche NW, Munn RJ, Gardner MB (1986) Seroepidemiologic survey of captive Old World primates for antibodies to human and simian retroviruses, and isolation of lentivirus from sooty mangabeys (*Cercocebus atys*). *Int J Cancer* 38: 563–575
23. Prince AM, Moor-Jankowski J, Eichberg JW, Schellekens H, Mauler RF, Girard M, Goudall J (1988) Chimpanzees and AIDS research. *Nature* 333: 523
24. Saag MS, Hahn BH, Gibbons J, Li Y, Parks ES, Parks WP, Shaw GM (1988) Extensive variation of human immunodeficiency virus type-1 in vivo. *Nature* 334: 440–444
25. Fisher AG, Ensoli B, Looney D, Rose A, Gallo RC, Saag MS, Shaw GM, Hahn BH, Wong-Staal F (1988) Biologically diverse molecular variants within a single HIV-1 isolate. *Nature* 334: 444–447

The need for animal experimentation in drug and vaccine development against tropical diseases

A. MONCAYO
World Health Organization Geneva, Switzerland

Introduction

The appropriate use of animals for biomedical research has been of concern to the World Health Organization (WHO) in the last decade and its highest governing body, the World Health Assembly, has approved relevant resolutions in 1975 and 1976 urging member states to promote programmes for breeding animals, notably simians, to be used in biomedical and veterinary research. The above resolutions also requested that WHO be responsible for the production of guidelines for adequate and ethical use of experimental animals and a publication on Guiding Principles was issued in 1985.

The UNDP/WORLD BANK/WHO Special Programme for Research and Training in Tropical Diseases (TDR) whose aim is the development of new drugs and vaccines for the control of six major tropical diseases (malaria, schistosomiasis, filariasis, trypanosomiasis – both African sleeping sickness and Chagas' Disease – leishmaniasis and leprosy) has sponsored research projects where animals are used in compliance with the above principles.

Some examples of the achievements in drug and vaccine research and development through animal experimentation sponsored by TDR are *Ivermectin*, a microfilaricidal effective against onchocerciasis and lymphatic filariasis and *Mefloquine*, an efficacious drug against multiresistant falciparum malaria. Inbred armadillos have been necessary for *M.leprae* culture in leprosy vaccine development projects and simians are being used to test immunoprotective antigens to develop a safe and effective malaria vaccine.

Screening systems using mice and monkeys are being used to select compounds with activity against African trypanosomiasis, Chagas' disease and leishmaniasis and to understand the mechanisms responsible for the pathogenesis of these diseases.

Background

In 1975 the World Health Assembly (WHA), the governing body of the World

S. Garattini (ed.), The Importance of Animal Experimentation for Safety and Biomedical Research, 163–171.

Health Organization (WHO), approved a resolution in which Member States were urged to cooperate in establishing colonies for breeding simians to ensure their long-term availability for research purposes [1].

In 1976 the WHA approved another resolution in which Member Countries were requested to strengthen the development of this resource and to support programmes for production of non-human primates in breeding colonies and/or in special reserves. At the same time the Director General of WHO was requested to make expert advise available to countries with regard to conservation, breeding, supply and utilization of non-human primates. On that occasion the Assembly requested that the World Health Organization provide leadership in the preparation of international guidelines on the appropriate use of simians in biomedical research [2].

Ethical principles

The Council for International Organizations of Medical Sciences (CIOMS), an international non-governmental organization established jointly by WHO and UNESCO in 1949, after extensive international and interdisciplinary consultations, issued the 'International Guiding Principles for Biomedical Research involving Animals' where basic ethical principles on this subject are stated [3]. They can be summarized as follows:

1. The advancement of biological knowledge and the development of new means for the protection of health requires experimentation on live animals of a wide variety of species. Experiments with animals should only be carried out after due consideration is given to their relevance for human and animal health and they should be undertaken on a minimum number of animals required to obtain statistically significant results. The animal species should be adequate to the nature and foreseeable outcome of the experiment.

2. Investigators and related personnel should always treat animals as sentient and consider their proper care and the minimalization of distress and pain as ethical imperatives. It should be assumed that procedures that would cause pain to human beings cause pain in other vertebrates and in particular painful procedures on unanesthetized animals should be avoided.

3. The best possible living conditions for experimental animals should be provided and their adequate care should be ensured by veterinary and other properly trained personnel.

This publication also features special provisions concerning acquisition, transportation, housing, nutrition, record keeping and monitoring of experimental animals.

The UNDP/WORLD BANK/WHO Special Programme for Research and Training in Tropical Diseases (TDR)

The TDR Programme, launched in 1976, is an international venture co-sponsored by three United Nations Agencies that has two interrelated objectives, namely:

– To develop new methods for the prevention, diagnosis and treatment of selected tropical diseases, methods that should be applicable, acceptable and affordable by developing countries, that require minimal skills or supervision and that are easily integrated into the health services of these countries; and

– To strengthen, through training in biomedical and social sciences and through support to institutions, the capability of developing countries to undertake the research required to develop these new disease control techniques.

The TDR Programme is a coordinated effort to mobilise the resources of modern science towards the development of new tools for the control of six major tropical diseases: malaria, filariasis (including onchocerciasis), schistosomiasis, trypanosomiasis (both African sleeping sickness and Chagas' disease), leishmaniasis and leprosy. These diseases were chosen because of their major impact on public health, because of the inadequacy of current methods used for attack and the likelihood that research could contribute to better control.

The TDR Programme is unique in that it has recruited into its worldwide network the best available scientific experts on different disciplines related to the above diseases, who are in charge of the definition of research priorities – the Scientific Working Groups. The Steering Committees are responsible for the detailed review of research projects sponsored by TDR that are conductive to the accomplishment of the Programme objectives.

More than sixty 'products' for improved diagnosis, treatment and control of the target diseases have resulted from research sponsored by TDR, including diagnostic tests, defined antigens for vaccine development, drugs and vector control tools [4]. Animal experimentation has been crucial for the development of these 'products'. Some examples are given in the following sections.

Animal experimentation for drug development

IVERMECTIN: a macrocyclic lactone antibiotic derived from *Streptomyces avermitilis*, an effective microfilaricidal agent

Lymphatic filariasis ('elephantiasis') and onchocerciasis ('river blindness') are among the eight human filarial infections of interest to TDR in view of their public health and clinical importance.

LYMPHATIC FILARIASIS is caused by *Wuchereria bancrofti, Brugia malayi* and *Brugia timori* and is transmitted by mosquitos of *Aedes*, *Anopheles* and *Culex* species.

The disease is endemic in many tropical and subtropical countries of Africa, Central and South America and Asia covering an area inhabited by 2700 million people or 56% of the world's population. Over 900 million people are at direct risk of infection and more than 90 million are actually infected [5].

The main clinical feature of the acute stage is the inflammation of lymph nodes and lymphatic vessels of the extremities. Elephantiasis and hydrocele are the clinical manifestations of the chronic stage.

ONCHOCERCIASIS is caused by *Onchocerca volvulus* and is transmitted by *Simulium* blackflies.

The disease is endemic in 26 African tropical countries, 6 Latin American countries (Brazil, Colombia, Ecuador, Guatemala, Mexico and Venezuela) and 2 Eastern Mediterranean countries (Sudan and Democratic Yemen) with a total population of 585 million, of whom 85 million are at risk of infection, 17.6 are actually infected and 336,000 have become blind as a result of the disease [6].

The treatment of the filarial diseases is chemotherapy (diethylcarbamazine - DEC - and suramin) and surgery for the chronic manifestations such as elephantiasis and hydrocele. However the drugs that have been used produce severe side effects, notably Mazzotti's reaction, a generalized allergic attack that requires specialized medical care. In addition no suitable drug has been available for mass treatment.

The development of a better drug, with no side effects and appropriate for mass treatment has been a high priority for the TDR Programme. Setting up a coordinated world-wide network of drug screening systems was a major undertaking made possible because of the international character of TDR.

In fact, with the exception of the small number of assays being used by the pharmaceutical industry to test their own compounds, few screens were available to test compounds for antifilarial activity. The TDR Programme created screening centers to test promising compounds against the parasites causing the above diseases.

The use of different animal species to conduct the experiments is obligatory for these initial steps in the drug development process, as can be seen in the following summary.

Using the above screening network it was possible to test more than 12,000 compounds.

These screening activities have yielded three compounds that have proved active against filarial infections and have reached the stage of trials in humans: Ivermectin developed by Merck, Sharp and Dohme, Rahway, NJ, USA and two compounds, CGP 6140 and CGP 20376 developed by Ciba-geigy, Basel, Switzerland.

Table 1. Screening systems for compounds with antifilarial activity. 1980–88

Screening system	Animal used	Purpose	Countries
Primary	Rodents	General Antifilarial activity	Germany Japan UK USA
Secondary	Rodents Cats Dogs	Dosage and side-effect determination	Australia Germany Malasia UK
Tertiary	Cattle Monkeys	Specific activity against human filarial parasites	Germany UK USA

Community trials are now being carried out with good therapeutic results and few side-effects in Cameroon, Guatemala, Liberia, Nigeria, and Malawi, involving a total of some 70,000 persons.

MEFLOQUINE: an effective compound against multiresistant falciparum malaria

Malaria is caused by a parasite of the genus *Plasmodium* of which four species infect humans: *P.falciparum, P. vivax, P.ovale,* and *P.malariae.* The falciparum or malignant tertian malaria is the most dangerous form of the disease.

Transmission of the infection occurs when sexual parasite forms are ingested by female mosquitos of the genus *Anopheles.* The parasite undergoes sporogony transformation in the mosquito and reaches the stage of sporozoite, the infected form that is inoculated by the mosquito into the susceptible human host.

Malaria transmission occurs in 102 countries: about 2,700 million people or 56% of the world population live in areas endemic for malaria. In 1984, the latest year for which figures are available, 5.3 million cases of malaria were reported to WHO [7].

The malaria situation in the world has not improved in the past 15 years. In most parts of the endemic countries, particularly in rural areas undergoing social, economic and ecological changes, the disease is becoming more frequent. In Africa rapid and unplanned urbanization has led to an increasing incidence of the disease in cities. In Brazil, agricultural and mining exploitation projects have produced an upsurge of malaria cases in the north western states of that country.

In addition to the worldwide increased incidence of the disease, the appearance of resistance to chloroquine has become a major obstacle for malaria control. *Plasmodium falciparum* resistance to chloroquine was first described in Columbia and Thailand in the 1960s and since then it has spread to other areas of the Americas and Asia, and more recently, to Africa.

Mefloquine, a 4-quinolinemethanol, has been the only new antimalarial to be clinically tested in more than 30 years. It is a potent blood schizontocide, active against multiresistant falciparum malaria, that has been developed by the concerted efforts of the Walter Reed Army Institute for Medical Research (WRAIR), Washington, DC, Hoffmann-La Roche and Co., Basel, Switzerland and TDR.

The drug has now been registered for use as a monosubstance in France and Switzerland and as a triple combination (mefloquine/sulfadoxine/pyrimethamine) in Brazil, Burma, Colombia, Ecuador, France, New Zealand, the Philippines, Surinam, Switzerland, Thailand and Zimbabwe.

Before the above compound reached the level of clinical trials it had to go through screening systems in animals of different species, namely rodents, dogs and monkeys.

Animal experimentation for vaccine development

LEPROSY VACCINE

Leprosy, or Hansen's disease, is a chronic communicable disease caused by *Mycobacterium leprae* which is believed to enter the body through the upper respiratory tract or the skin. The clinical manifestations of the disease include a broad spectrum of signs and symptoms that range from subclinical infection to severe disfiguring disease. The most currently accepted clinical classification of leprosy distinguishes five forms that extend from *tuberculoid leprosy* (TT) with few lesions, to *lepromatous leprosy* (LL) with varied lesions. Intermediate forms between these two poles are: *borderline tuberculoid* (BT), *mid-borderline* (BB) and *borderline lepromatous leprosy* (BL). The most contagious forms of multibacillary leprosy are BB, BL, and LL. These clinical forms are also related to the degree of a patient's immunity to *M.leprae* which is very strong at the tuberculoid end of the spectrum and practically nonexistent at the lepromatous pole.

Skin lesions associated with loss of sensitivity are common and range in severity from hypopigmented patches to thickening and folding of the skin that confers the 'leonine' aspect to the face. Loss of peripheral sensitivity in the limbs results in unnoticed ulcers and burns and the involvement of nerve axons causes muscle weakness and atrophy with the subsequent limb deformity.

Leprosy is common in Asia, Africa and Latin America: an estimated 1,600 million people or one third of the world's population, live in areas where prevalence rates for leprosy are 1/1000 inhabitants or greater. The total number of leprosy patients in the world is estimated at 12 to 15 million [8].

The currently recommended treatment is based on multidrug therapy (MDT) with rifampicin, dapsone and clofazimine which has the advantage of shorter treatment courses and lower probability of development of drug resistance.

The prevention of this disease was made possible by the development of immunoprophylactic regimens based on the production of *M.leprae* in armadillos. Two extensive trials using killed *M.leprae* vaccines are now under way in Malawi and Venezuela involving some 30,000 individuals. Results on efficacy of the vaccine are expected in five years' time in view of the long incubation period of the disease and its relatively low incidence rates.

The use of the armadillo as a source of *M.leprae* started in 1971. This animal was chosen for various reasons including its low body temperature (30°–36°C), life span of 12–15 years and the fact that it has a regular offspring of monozygous quadruplets which makes it possible to replicate experiments with genetically identical animals [9].

M.leprae from infected armadillos has been produced by a network of five breeding colonies that are maintained in the USA, the UK and Venezuela. A central bank in the UK processes infected tissues of some 300 armadillos and purifies the bacillus material for vaccine preparations and skin tests for the above mentioned trials in humans.

In addition, after the recent cloning and expression of the *M.leprae* genome in *E.coli*, it will be possible to obtain defined relevant antigens for vaccine production through recombinant DNA technology or protein synthesis [10].

MALARIA VACCINE

Malaria vaccines for human use will be based on plasmodial antigens from different stages of the life cycle of the parasite, which stimulate protective immune response in the host. The antigens that are of potential interest for vaccine development are present in the following parasite stages:

Sporozoites. Parasite infective forms present in the blood stream. A vaccine effective against this infective stage of the malaria parasite would prevent the host becoming infected and developing parasitemia. It would also prevent infection to mosquitos.

Asexual blood-stages. Schizonts and merozoites of the parasite present in the blood. A vaccine against these stages of the parasite would restrict parasite multiplication in the host blood stream and reduce morbidity. It would not prevent infection to mosquitos.

Sexual-stages. Gametes present in the mosquito. A vaccine against these stages would induce host antibodies that would be ingested by the mosquito, block parasite development towards the infective sporozoite stage in the mosquito midgut and block transmission of the disease in the community.

The most effective vaccine might be a combination of antigens from more than one stage of the parasite's life cycle.

The identification and characterization of the above antigens, as well as

Table 2. Animal models in three major tropical diseases

Disease	Animal species	Clinical and laboratory findings
African Trypanosomiasis		
	Mouse	Early and late stages Central nervous system (CNS) involvement (*T.b.brucei*)
	Vervet monkey (*Cercopithecus*)	Early and encephalitic stages (*T.b.rhodesiense*)
	Sheep	Encephalitic stage (*T.b.brucei*)
	Rat	Chronic stage with CNS and heart involvement (*T.b.gambiense*)
American Trypanosomiasis		
	Mouse	Acute and chronic phases with myocardial lesions
	Rabbit	Acute and chronic phases with myocardial and digestive involvement
	Dog	Acute and chronic phases with myocardial involvement
	Monkey (*Coebus*)	Acute and chronic phases with myocardial lesions
Leishmaniasis		
	Hamster	Cutaneous and visceral forms
	Mouse	Old world cutaneous form (*L.major*)
	Monkey (*Aoutus*)	Old world visceral form (*L.donovani*)
	Monkey (*Saimiri* and *Callithrix*)	New world cutaneous form (*L.b.brasiliensis*)

the cloning of the parasite genetic material that encode for them, has been made possible by the extensive use of laboratory animals, namely mice. Their immunoprotective capacity has been assessed using non-human primates, a necessary step before any clinical trial to test the effectiveness of candidate malaria vaccine [11].

The primate species known to be most suitable for this purpose (*Aotus* and *Saimiri* species of New World monkeys) are not classified as endangered, vulnerable or rare but their supply is limited. Therefore, for ethical and economic reasons it has to be ensured that experiments using non-human primates are fully justified and designed to yield unequivocal results.

Animal experimentation to understand disease pathogenesis

The use of animals of a variety of species to understand disease pathogenic mechanisms is another example that illustrates their irreplaceable role in the advance of biomedical research.

Three examples of tropical diseases in which a better understanding of pathogenesis has been gained by the development of animal models are African trypanosomiasis (sleeping sickness), American trypanosomiasis (Chagas' disease) and leishmaniasis. A summary of major clinical and laboratory findings of animal models for the above diseases is presented above [12,13].

References

1. World Health Assembly (1975) Resolution WHA-28.83, *Handbook of Resolutions and Decisions of the World Health Assembly and the Executive Board, Volume II*, 1973–1984, p 127, World Health Organization, Geneva
2. World Health Assembly (1976) Resolution WHA-29.67, *Handbook of Resolutions and Decisions of the World Health Assembly and the Executive Board, Volume II*, 1973–1984, p 128, World Health Organization, Geneva
3. C.I.O.M.S. (1985) *International Guiding Principles for Biomedical Research Involving Animals* CIOMS, Geneva, pp 17–21
4. UNDP/WORLD BANK/WHO Special Programme for Research and Training in Tropical Diseases (1987) *Tropical Disease Research: A global Partnership* pp 10–11, World Health Organization, Geneva
5. Idem p 63
6. Idem pp 63–64
7. Idem pp 19–21
8. Idem pp 115–116
9. Kirchheimer WF and Storrs EE (1971) Attempts to establish the Armadillo (*Dasypus novemcinctus*, Linn.) as a model for the study of Leprosy. *International Journal of Leprosy* 39: 3, pp 693–702

10 Young RA *et al.* (1985) Genes for the major protein antigens of the Leprosy parasite *Mycobacterium leprae*. *Nature* 316: 450–452

11. Patarroyo ME *et al.* (1987) Induction of protective immunity against experimental infection with malaria using synthetic peptides. *Nature* 328: 629–632
12. WHO/TDR (1985) Report of the Steering Committees of the Scientific Working Group on African Trypanosomiasis, TDR/TRY/SC-SWG 81–85/85. 3: 30
13. WHO/TDR (1984) Report of the Scientific Working Group on the development and evaluation of Animal Models for Chagas' disease, TDR/IMMCHA-AMOD/84.3

USE OF ANIMALS FOR SAFETY REASONS

Toxicology: Role of *in vivo* studies in establishing mechanisms of toxicity

JAMES W. BRIDGES
The Robens Institute of Industrial and Environmental Health and Safety, University of Surrey, Guildford, Surrey, UK

Introduction

Mechanisms of toxicity studies are important for a number of purposes [1], namely:

- to rationalise dose-response relationships for particular toxic effects, including the establishment of a clear basis for the threshold dose;
- to assist in the extrapolation of findings from one animal species to another;
- to characterise the likely principal factors influencing the severity of toxic effects;
- to provide a better basis for structure activity predictions;
- to increase the understanding of basic biology.

Many chemicals are selectively toxic to a particular cell type/organ (Table 1). An important aspect of investigating mechanisms of toxicity is to seek of this target selectivity. Both *in vivo* and *in vitro* studies are necessary in order to elucidate the underlying mechanisms of toxicity of each chemical (see Fig. 1). The starting point for most investigations of mechanisms of toxicity is sound *in vivo* findings on the target site and nature of toxicity preferably

Table 1. Examples of 'cell type' specific toxic effects

Target	Chemical
2-Bromoethylamine	Renal medulla
Puromycin aminonucleoside	Renal glomerulus
Paraquat	Type 2 cells of lung
4-Ipomeanol	Lung clara cells
Tri-o-cresylphosphate	Nerve long axon
Triethyl tin chloride	Brain white matter
Thalidomide	Foetus
Gentamycin	Ear
Chloroquine	Eye
Benzene	Bone marrow
α Naphthylisocyanate	Liver (jaundice)

S. Garattini (ed.), The Importance of Animal Experimentation for Safety and Biomedical Research, 175–184.

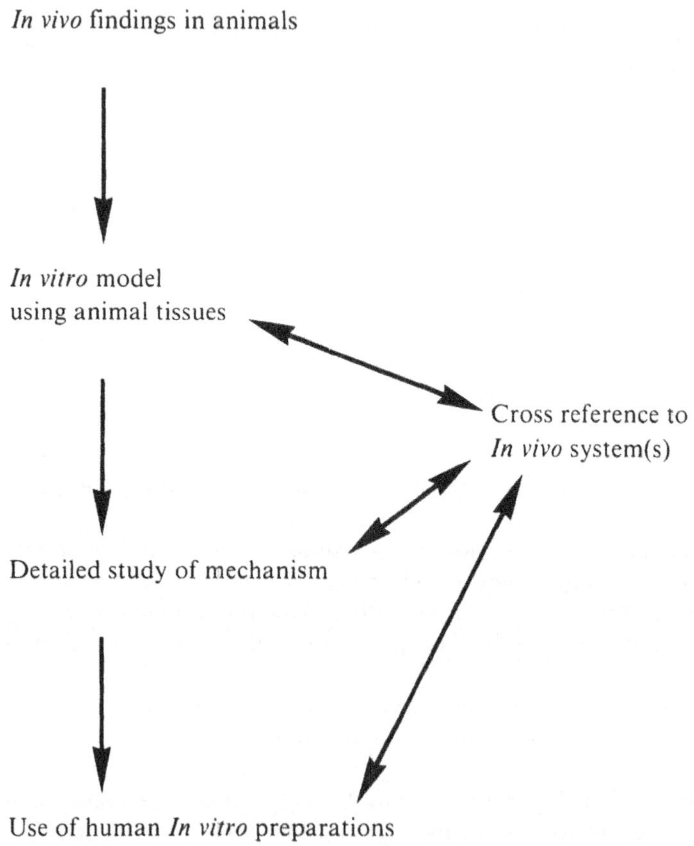

Fig. 1. Role of *In vivo* and *In vitro* studies in investigating mechanisms of toxicity

coupled with good information on the relationship between dose (or, better still, target organ concentrations) and toxic response [2].

Using such information *in vitro* models can be developed [2]. Normally these would be intact cell preparations or tissue cultures or cell fractions derived from the target cell type. If the toxic effect is acute involving a single, relatively non-specialised cell type the prospects of replicating the crucial elements of the *in vivo* toxicity *in vitro* are good. If, however, the toxic effect is a slowly developing one and/or more than one cell type or more than one tissue is involved then replication *in vitro* may prove to be very difficult, if not impossible, without a major advance in cell technology. For slowly developing lesions and for toxicity mechanisms involving different cell types or tissues, the bulk of the work on the elucidation of mechanisms typically needs to be conducted *in vivo*. (Table 2 provides examples of chemically induced lesions which at least at present we are not capable of replicating *in vitro*).

The purpose of this article is by use of a few examples from the work

Table 2. Types of toxicity difficult to replicate *in vitro*

A.	Lesions involving specialised cell types
–	Neurotoxicity
–	Ototoxicity
–	Diarrhoea
–	Inflammation
–	Some forms of enzyme induction
B.	Lesions which are slow in onset
–	Hypertension
–	Tumours
–	Arteriosclerosis
–	Demyelination
–	Chronic asthma
–	Teratogenicity
–	Ulceration
C.	Lesions involving cell-cell or tissue-tissue interactions
–	Hormonal, eg: various organ changes due to altered hormone status
–	Immunological, eg: allergic response
–	Neurological, eg: delayed neurotoxicity with muscular atrophy

of our own laboratory to illustrate the current contribution of *in vivo* studies to investigate ions of the mechanisms of toxicity. However, the illustrations do also emphasise the enormous value of suitable *in vitro* preparations in elucidating how chemicals mediate their toxicity. The common theme among these examples is that the initial effect for each type of chemical involves the liver. The rationale for selecting liver effects is two-fold: firstly the liver is the most frequent target site in animal models for chemically mediated cell damage, and secondly far more effort has been put into developing *in vitro* models for the liver than for any other organ.

Short-term effects

Drug metabolising enzyme changes

It is now well established that many lipophilic substrates of the principal oxidation enzyme system cytochrome P450 induce *in vivo de novo* synthesis of one or more isoforms of cytochrome P450 [3]. Chemicals may be classified according to the profile of isoforms of cytochrome P450 which they induce. The most common type of inducer is the co-called phenobarbitone type but a number of other types are known, including 3-methylcholanthrene type, pregnenolonecarbonitrile type, alcohol type, clofibrate type and benzodioxole type. For some types the induction appears to occur primarily or solely in liver, for others many organs are affected. The consequence of induction is normally enhanced removal of chemicals thus when considered in general terms it must be regarded as enhancing detoxication. However, in the course of metabolism by cytochrome P450 and other drug metabolising enzymes, highly toxic intermediates can be produced; consequently for certain chemicals selective induction among the drug metabolising enzymes results in greatly enhanced toxicity [4].

It is therefore important to establish: which chemicals induce the specific drug metabolising enzymes (particularly in man and environmentally important species) and the toxicological implications of prolonged induction. It is obviously impossible to assess induction for every combination of chemicals in every species. However, many of the important toxicological issues may be resolved once an understanding of the mechanism(s) of induction has been attained.

Establishing which drug metabolising enzymes are induced in which tissues and the dose response relationship for the induction initially requires *in vivo* investigations. Once this information has been obtained, *in vitro* studies are very valuable to examine the details of the progression of cellular changes leading to induction and also the processes of recovery when the inducer is withdrawn. Because induction requires *de novo* protein synthesis an intact cell system and between 12 h and several days depending on the type of inducer, are needed. Drug metabolising enzyme activity tends to fall off rapidly with time particularly in dividing cultures as does sensitivity to most types of inducer. As a consequence induction, with the exception of the 3-methylcholanthrene type inducers, can at present only be investigated properly in primary maintenance cultures [5].

Most preparations only have a useful lifetime of up to five days after the tissue has been removed from an animal. Nonetheless, within this period it is possible to replicate the key features of the induction process for phenobarbitone type, 3-methylcholanthrene type [6] and clofibrate type inducers [7] in primary maintenance cultures of rat and mouse hepatocytes. Interestingly in contrast to phenobarbitone and 3-methylcholanthrene types, clofibrate type inducers are not effective in hepatocytes from man, marmoset or guinea pig [8]; this resembles the *in vivo* situation.

Because the induction process can be replicated *in vitro* very considerable progress has been made in establishing the mechanism(s) of induction of these three types of inducer, particularly the 3-methylcholanthrene type. This has led to an increased appreciation of the long term consequences of induction of this type and established a rational basis for assessing the effects of combinations of such chemicals [9].

Our laboratory has been particularly involved with the benzodioxole type inducing agents. Benzodioxoles, e.g.: safrole, myristicin and sasamol, are widely found in plant materials including many herbs and spices; they are used as insecticide synergists, e.g.: piperonylbutoxide, and the benzodioxole structure is also found in a number of drugs and industrial chemicals. When administered *in vivo* these chemicals act initially as potent inhibitors of cytochrome P450; this effect progressively gives way to induction of particular isoforms of cytochrome P450 which are at very low levels in control animals. The inhibitory effect of benzodioxoles can be readily demonstrated *in vitro*, both in intact hepatocytes and in hepatic microsomal fractions [10]. Use of these preparations has enabled us to identify the structural requirements for inhibition and characterise the mechanism of inhibition. This involves metabolic oxidation of the methylene carbon to a carbene which then binds tightly to the iron atom of cytochrome P450, thereby blocking further metabolism both of the benzodioxole concerned and of many other substrates of cytochrome P450, as follows:

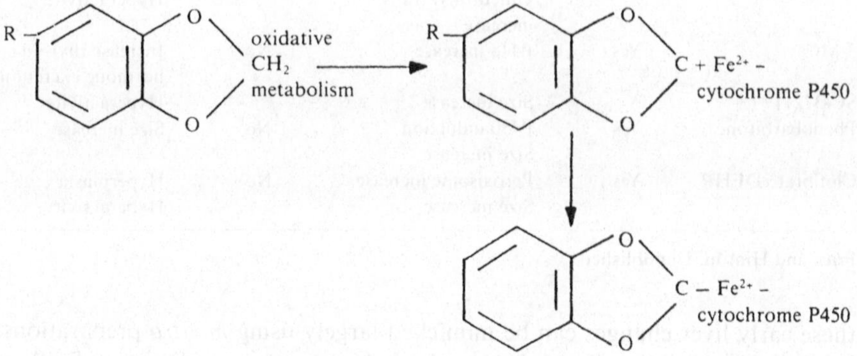

In vivo the structural requirements for induction of a particular isoform of cytochrome P450 (termed isoform D) in rat liver can be clearly defined, and this provides some clues to the mechanism likely to be involved [11]. Induction appears to be associated with the initial inhibition process. However, attempts to replicate the *in vivo* induction process *in vitro* have all been unsuccessful, indicating that the induction mechanism is more complex than that for phenobarbitone or methylcholanthrene. Possibly additional growth regulators or nutrients are required, or the process of induction by benzodioxoles may involve an additional cell type.

Since induction may be involved in the hepatotoxicity of benzodioxoles such as safrole and isosafrole it is important to identify the reasons for the differences between *in vivo* and *in vitro* studies [12]. This will require additional *in vivo* and *in vitro* research.

Effects of interactions between tissues – evidence of a liver thyroid axis

There are increasing numbers of reports of an association between the ability of non-genotoxic chemicals to cause liver tumours in rates and effects on the thyroid gland (see Table 3). It should be noted that most of these chemicals are inducers of both oxidation and conjugation hepatic drug metabolising enzymes. The thyroid changes observed range from increased hyperactivity to tumours. *In vivo* studies have indicated that early liver changes occur before any changes are observable in either thyroid function or morphology. Although

Table 3. Effects of various chemicals on the liver and thyroid

Compound	Liver		Thyroid	
	Carcin-ogenic	Short term change	Carcin-ogenic	Short term change
Toxaphene	Yes	DM enzymes increase	Yes	Not reported
Dieldrin/Aldrin	Yes	DM enzymes increase. Glucuronyl trans. increase	Yes	Hyperplasia and hyperactivity
PCBs and PBBs	Yes	DM enzymes increase. Glucuronyl trans. increase	No	Hyperplasia Hyperactivity
3-MC	Yes	P448 increase	No	Increase thyroid hormone excretion
SC-37211	?	Size increase	?	Hyperactivity
Phenobarbitone	Yes	P450 induction Size increase	No	Size increase
Clofibrate DEHP	Yes	Peroxisome increase. Size increase	No	Hyperplasia Hyperactivity

Price and Hinton, Unpublished.

these early liver changes can be mimicked largely using *in vitro* preparations, i.e.: primary maintenance cultures of rat hepatocytes, preliminary findings suggest that the thyroid changes cannot be reproduced using *in vitro* thyroid preparations. These data suggest that the liver changes actually provoke the thyroid changes. The observation may have some bearing on the aetiology of human thyroid cancer [13]. To pinpoint the likely mechanism involved detailed information is required on the sequence of changes taking place in each organ, the dose-response relationship and the blood chemistry profile with time (since the most likely route of interactions between liver and thyroid involves blood-borne substances). This information can only be derived *in vivo*. Several chemicals with rather different chemical structures and which cause different early profiles of hepatic change have been investigated. Each has been shown to cause common changes in blood chemistry, namely a large fall in thyroxine (T4) levels, a slight fall in triiodothyronine (T3) and rise in the circulating levels of thyroid stimulating hormone (TSH). The thyroid gland's primary function is to produce T4 in response to the production of TSH by the pituitary gland: how can this activity be influenced by hepatic drug metabolising enzyme inducers administered chronically? Drug metabolising enzymes are involved in the metabolism of both foreign chemicals and endogenous substances, e.g.: circulating hormones. In the case of thyroxine a major route of inactivation is to thyroxine glucuronide, a biotransformation brought about by one of the drug metabolising enzymes which is readily induced (along with various cytochrome P450 isoforms), glucuronyl transferase. T4 is activated to triidothyronine which is then deactivated by progressive deiodination and formation of T3 glucuronide; these latter pathways also

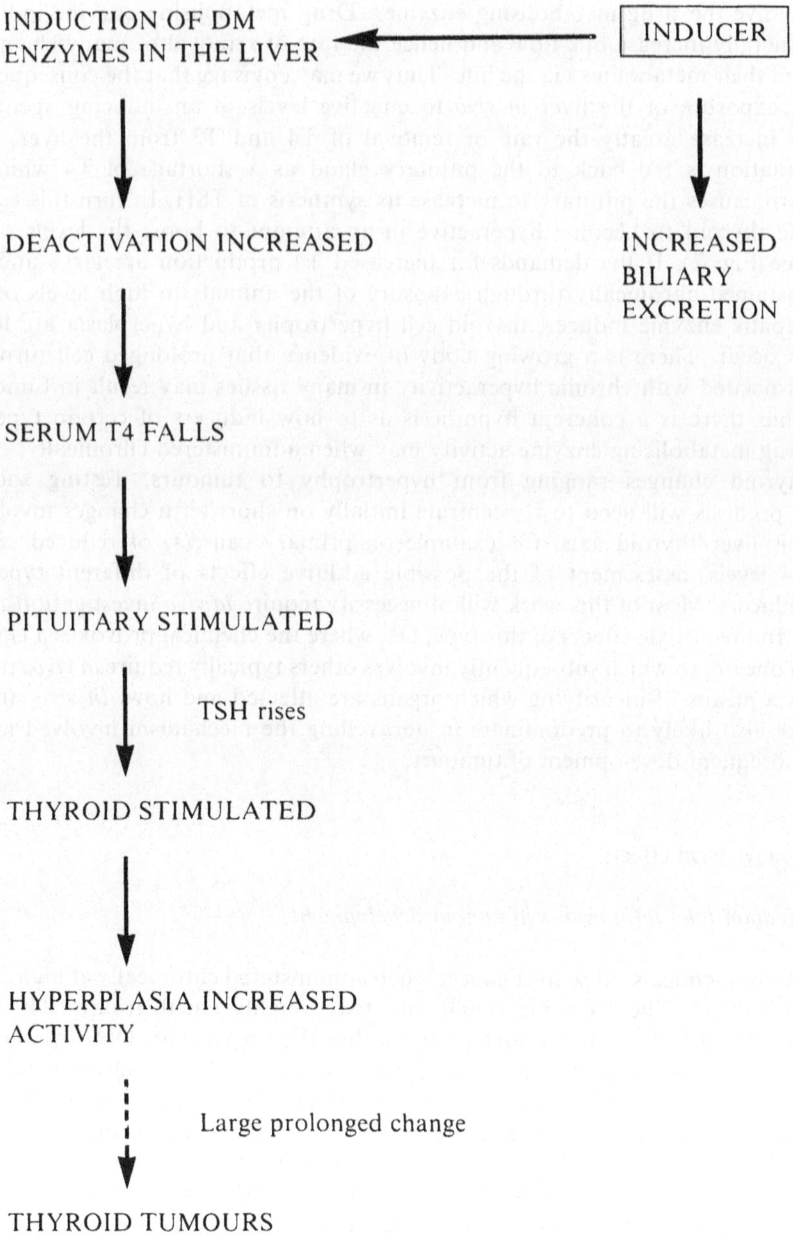

Fig. 2. Likely mechanisms involved in the liver/thyroid axis

involve the drug metabolising enzymes. Drug metabolising enzyme inducers generally increase bile flow and hence the rate of removal of many chemicals and their metabolites via the bile. Thus we may envisage that the consequences of exposure of the liver *in vivo* to effective levels of an inducing agent are to increase greatly the rate of removal of T4 and T3 from the liver. This situation is fed back to the pituitary gland as a shortage of T4 which in turn causes the pituitary to increase its synthesis of TSH. In turn this causes the thyroid to become hyperactive in an attempt to boost the levels of T4 (see Fig. 2). If the demands for increased T4 production are large and are sustained chronically through exposure of the animals to high levels of the hepatic enzyme inducer, thyroid cell hypertrophy and hyperplasia are likely to occur. There is a growing body of evidence that prolonged cell turnover associated with chronic hyperactivity in many tissues may result in tumours. Thus there is a coherent hypothesis as to how inducers of certain types of drug metabolising enzyme activity may when administered chronically, cause thyroid changes ranging from hypertrophy to tumours. Testing such a hypothesis will need to concentrate initially on short term changes involving this liver/thyroid axis, for example on primary cause(s) of reduced serum T4 levels, assessment of the possible additive effects of different types of inducers. Most of this work will of necessity require *in vivo* investigations.

Indirect toxic effects of this type, i.e.: where the chemical provokes a change in one organ which subsequently involves others typically require *in vivo* studies as a means of identifying which organs are affected and how. *In vivo* studies are also likely to predominate in unravelling the mechanism involved in the subsequent development of tumours.

Longer term effects

Medium-long term events in tumour development

Many chemicals cause liver cancer when administered chronically at high doses to rodents. These chemicals fall into two roughly equal groups. The characteristic feature of the first group is that they react with DNA of the cell (genes) either directly or through the formation of a reactive metabolite (produced by one or more of the drug metabolising enzymes). In dividing cell populations there is a prospect of the altered genes being transferred to a new cell before they can be repaired/replaced. If this occurs a new cell type - a mutated cell - is produced. It is believed that certain types of mutated cells in particular circumstances may ultimately grow at the expense of surrounding normal cells, thereby resulting in adenomas and carcinomas [14]. Chemicals which are thought to cause cancer by this mechanism are called genotoxic. Such chemicals are, with few exceptions, believed to pose a carcinogenic risk to man and many believe that there may be no threshold dose below which carcinogenicity cannot occur. Many of their early effects but not yet the later ones can be reproduced *in vitro*.

The second group of hepatocarcinogens initially at least changes which do not directly involve the genetic elements of the cell and are therefore described as non-genotoxic. This title covers a miscellancy of mechanisms. It is necessary to identify the mechanism involved for economically important chemicals in order to provide a rationale for extrapolation of findings from life-time studies in animals to the actual human exposure situation.

One distinct group of such chemicals (known generally as peroxisome proliferators) can be characterised by the fact that among the early hepatic effects they produce in rodents (i.e.: up to 3 days) are enlarged liver cells, cell division, peroxisome proliferation, induction of a particular isoform of cytochrome P450 involved in lauric acid metabolism (P452), reduction in cellular thiols and a loss of cellular glucose-6-phosphatase activity. With the exception of the last two changes these effects can be replicated in primary maintenance cultures of rat hepatocytes [7]. It is notable that these effects are also seen *in vivo* in mice, but not guinea pigs or marmosets; this species difference also holds true *in vitro*. Although *in vivo* studies indicate a very good correlation in rats between ability of chemicals to produce peroxisome proliferation and their hepatocarcinogenic potential there is as yet no firm mechanistic basis on which to explain this correlation. Following peroxisome proliferation in rodents it has been established that a number of other changes occur: these include single cell necrosis and a build up of lipofuscin – a cellular product associated usually with oxidative damage to the lipid membranes of subcellular organelles, e.g.: mitochondria and endoplasmic reticulum [16]. Whether and how these later changes are linked to the development of tumours is unclear [17]. As yet the technology for primary maintenance culture of hepatocytes is not sufficiently developed to allow investigation of any of the longer term effects of chemicals. Consequently studies of the links between peroxisome proliferation and oxidative damage and between both types of change and tumour development must rely heavily on further *in vivo* investigations.

Conclusions

With few exceptions *in vivo* studies have and continue to play a crucial role in establishing mechanisms of toxicity. As methods improve for preserving cells and tissues from various target tissues in a state more resembling that *in vivo*, the emphasis in unravelling mechanisms is likely to shift more to *in vitro* preparations. Nonetheless, *in vivo* methods are likely to be necessary for the foreseeable future both for initial characterisation of toxic lesions and to confirm *in vitro* findings. Reproducing *in vitro* toxic phenomena which are of slow onset and/or involve interactions between different tissues is a particularly challenging task. One area where progress is crucial to more effective and widespread use of *in vitro* preparations for mechanism studies is the mimicking of pharmacokinetic phenomena, particularly absorption, distribution and excretion kinetics.

References

1. Bernard S (Ed) *Mechanisms of cell injury: implications for human health.* J Wiley, Chichester (1987)
2. Bridges JW, Chasseaud LF, Cohen GC, Walker C (1983) Application of pharmacokinetics to toxicity evaluation, p 30–67 In: M Balls, RJ Riddell and AN Worden (Eds) *Animals and alternatives in toxicity testing.* Academic Press, London
3. Estabrook RW, Lindenlaub E (Eds) *The induction of drug metabolism.* FK Schattaver Verlag, Stuttgart (1978)
4. Snyder R, Parke DV, Kocsis JJ, Jollow DJ, Gibson GG, Witmer CM (Eds) *Biological reactive intermediates.* Parts A and B, Plenum Press, New York (1982)
5. Bridges JW (1981) The use of isolated hepatocytes in assessing chemically induced toxicity, p 125–144 In: JW Gorrod (Ed) *Toxicity testing of pharmaceuticals and other products.* Taylor and Francis, London
6. Fry JR, Wiebkin P, Bridges JW (1980) 7 ethoxy-O-deethylation induction by phenobarbitone and 1,2 benzanthracene in primary maintenance cultures of adult hepatocytes. *Biochem Pharmacol* 29: 577–581
7. Mitchell A, Elcombe CR, Bridges JW (1985) Factors influencing peroxisome proliferation in cultured rat hepatocytes. *Archives Toxicol* 55: 239–246
8. Mitchell A (1985) PhD Thesis, University of Surrey
9. Poland A, Knutson JC (1982) 2,3,7,8 tetra-chlorodibenzo-p-dioxin and related halogenated aromatic hydrocarbons: examination of the mechanisms of toxicity. *Ann Rev Pharmacol and Toxicol* 22: 517–544
10. Elcombe CR, Bridges JW, Gray TJR, Nimmo-Smith RH, Netter KJ (1975) Studies on the interaction of safrole with rat hepatic microsomes. *Biochem Pharmacol* 24: 1427–1433
11. Fennel TR, Bridges JW (1979) Structure activity relationship for safrole type P450 induction. *Biochem Soc Transac* 7: 1104–1106
12. Bridges JW, Fennell TR (1982) The relationship between metabolism and toxicity of benzodioxoles, p 881–893 In: R Snyder, DV Parke, JJ Kocsis, DJ Jollow, GG Gibson and GM Witmer (Eds) *Biological reactive intermediates.* Plenum Press, New York
13. Hinton RH, Mitchell FE, Mann A, Chescoe D, Price SC, Nunn A, Grasso P, Bridges JW (1986) Effect of phthalic acid esters on the liver and thyroid. *Environ Health Perspectives* 70: 195–210
14. Williams GM, Dunkel VC, Ray VA (Eds) *Cellular systems for toxicity testing.* Annals New York Academy of Sciences, Vol 407 (1983)
15. Mitchell FE, Price SC, Hinton RH, Grasso P, Bridges JW (1985) Time and dose response study of effects on rats of the plasticiser di(2-ethylhexyl)phthalate. *Toxicol Pharmacol* 81: 371–392
16. Bridges JW (1986) Use of toxicity data – a case study of di-(2-ethylhexyl)phthalate, p 233–246 In: ML Richardson (Ed) *Toxic hazard assessment of chemicals.* Royal Society of Chemistry, London

Necessity of animal experiments for the safety evaluation and necessary regular consequences for public health

JEAN-ROGER CLAUDE and HÉLÈNE DUTERTRE-CATELLA
Laboratory of Toxicoloy, Faculty of Pharmacy, Paris, France

In the course of the ages, man's safety in his way of life has undergone many changes. Progressively the risks due to contact with or absorption of xenobiotics have increased for several reasons:

- the native environment of man is not necessarily propitious, as in J.J. Rousseau's philosophy or in the finalist theories, and now contains many toxic compounds, not known to earlier generations. Industrial and technical progress has increased their quantity.
- Men eat and drink and try to improve both the quantity (pesticides) and quality (additives of their food).
- Men work and can come into contact with occupational compounds, responsible for troubles and diseases.
- Men take care of themselves and use drugs with great efficacy, but also with high toxicity. This is true for animals too.
- Men come under 'society' influences, related to fashion (cosmetics) or to harmful habits (tobacco, alcohol, narcotics...).

Moreover, all human activities are likely to modify the quality of the environment with consequences on animal and vegetable life (toxicity on ecosystems), and finally also on human health.

For all these reasons, safety must be evaluated, this evaluation being vital for environmental or occupational protection against pollution, and for more and more compounds currently used as chemicals, pesticides, food additives, drugs, cosmetics and others.

Consequently, measures must be established to ensure this evaluation by the most suitable scientific procedures recognized by the international community. These measures, or regulations, will in many cases have regular support, because of governmental and administrative responsibilities for public health protection. Consumers themselves are calling for higher levels of safety for drugs, food additives, cosmetics and so forth, and the exposed workers and trade-unions for chemicals, pollutants, etc. The scientific tools available for attaining this high level of safety are not well known to the general public, and this tends to create equivocal attitudes toward some methods of investigation.

S. Garattini (ed.), The Importance of Animal Experimentation for Safety and Biomedical Research, 185–190.

What are, in consequence, the scientific approaches for suitable safety evaluation, for example, of chemicals, drugs, pesticides, food additives?

1. Physico-chemical evaluations are of great value for the detection of toxic products already known for their deleterious properties as a result of accidental observations on man or animals, or epidemiological studies. This is the case in occupational toxicology for exposure of workers to toxic gases, volatile substances, dusts or radioactivity. As a consequence in the field of regulations, the proposal of Maximal Allowable Concentrations (MAC) would define the limit of risk and serve as a basis for assessing the likelihood of occupational diseases. Environmental toxicology is in the same situation, with the possibility of determination of pollution indicators in air or water, with important consequences for the protection of public health. In the same way, for food additives, limitations of their use, depending on their hazardous properties, by the concept of Maximal Daily Intake, can be imposed in many cases, and the presence of toxic impurities in food, drugs etc., can be monitored.

This signifies that safety evaluation by a physico-chemical approach is one of the most satisfying approaches. Furthermore, improvements in the performance of the methods and in the sensitivity and specificity of available instruments now give extensive possibilities of investigations. Nevertheless, physico-chemical analysis is not suitable for elucidating the biological action(s) of toxic xenobiotics and is not able, alone, to demonstrate the toxic properties of new compounds (drugs for example) for living beings, or of well known compounds where new modes of toxicity are suspected.

Consequently, though physico-chemical analysis is obviously one of the best tools for the survey and the routine control of safety, but its use is clearly downstream of the discovery of the toxic potential of compounds where a biological approach is indispensable.

2. Direct evaluation on man has the considerable advantage of avoiding extrapolation from experimental models, but poses major ethical problems, leading to impossibility. As previously stated, accidental observations on man and animals, sometimes dating back many years (arsenic, carbon monoxide, cyanides, etc.), bring sufficient knowledge of the toxic properties of compounds, but it will be frequently necessary to perform studies with appropriate models to understand the mechanism or to reveal new and unknown toxic effects. The epidemiological approach is the most accurate for evaluation in man. Retrospective studies have demonstrated severe toxic effects in man in the last thirty years: teratogenic action of thalidomide, carcinogenic action of vinyl chloride, and especially in France – the responsibility of hexachlorophene in a collective intoxication of babies by a talcum powder, the surprising role still unexplained of bismuth compounds in lethal encephalitis and others. Such examples show the irreplaceable efficacy of retrospective studies when a fully unexpected toxic effect of a chemical or drug arises but also show the limits of this approach: the toxic effect becomes obvious a very long time after

the first cases of intoxication (sometimes many years), the attribution is difficult with many statistical biases, and the mechanism is not elucidated. Nevertheless, the usefulness of this approach through systems of drugs and toxico-surveillance is unquestionable.

Prospective studies, with suitable methodologies, are better tools for the epidemiological approach because many biases can be allowed for or avoided, but the time needed for such studies, their cost, and the ethical problems raised by the follow-up of populations including exposed or treated sub-samples versus controls limit their use. In environmental toxicology, these procedures are of great interest to point out the unexpected consequences of large and dramatic pollutions (Seveso, Bhopal, Chernobyl).

For drug studies, clinical trials, accepted by ethical committees, are necessary to evaluate efficacy, tolerance and side-effects. Nevertheless, preliminary data obtained from accurate models are ethically and practically compulsory prior to first administration to man, especially human volunteers.

3. Animal experiments have given the letters patent of nobility to safety evaluation. We have already mentioned the need for suitable 'models' for the evaluation of adverse effects and for their biological explanation (if possible). Historically, the animal model was the first to be used. The large-scale development of new chemicals, pesticides, food additives, drugs and other substances has extensively increased the use of animal experiments in toxicology for the following reasons:

– From a scientific point of view, it is obvious that a 'total' system is the sole suitable model to discover an adverse effect or a combination of adverse effects, linked to biological interactions. Evidently, this 'total' system is the animal *in toto*. Morphological lesions of tissues, cells or subcellular structures induce functional abnormalities with subsequent alterations of other tissues and functions with a possible lethal issue. Compared with the total animal, no other system is able to provide such a large amount of integrated information for the detection of adverse effects as well as for their mechanistic explanation.

– Concerning the protection of public health, governments, groupings of governments (EEC, OUA) international organizations in charge of health (WHO, JECFA) or economy (OECI) have, for their population or for all the world's peoples, the responsibility to ensure their protection as far as possible. This is why regulations or recommendations must be elaborated to protect populations against the greatest number of checked risks:

- Acute or chronic contact with harmful chemicals or pesticides, in occupational activities.
- Environmental pollution.
- Uncontrolled use of food additives, and contamination of food by toxic impurities, pesticides, etc.
- Use of drugs (for human or animals), cosmetics, etc. of questionable quality

and/or safety.

- Uncontrolled use of drugs.

At present, all the above mentioned authorities recognize that the highest level of safety for the populations exposed to these risks is obtained by toxicological requirements based upon animal experiments, because the conditions of exposure are flexible and comparable to the conditions of human exposure. Many people – scientists, jurists, politicians – have pronounced severe sentences against countries or companies responsible for the production or the use of toxic compounds without control or evaluation. Obviously such sentences are justified only if we recognize the necessity of using the best relevant model to ensure human safety, which is still the animal experiment. Imagine the justified general outcry if a collective drama occurred through a toxic compound that had not been experimentally evaluated!

Nevertheless, the question of extrapolation from animal to man must be considered. In a first approach, from a pragmatic point of view, we can bet that, if damages occurs in animals, it will also occur in man. In such a situation, it is reasonable to consider that the xenobiotic inducing the lesions is potentially toxic for man, with all the regular consequences. But now, a more scientific approach to this question is supported by toxico-pharmacokinetic and metabolic data. If it is possible to compare animal and human kinetic and metabolic parameters, the choice, for animal experiments, of the species most closely comparable to man powerfully supports extrapolation. This situation is especially true for long-term studies in animals, such as *in vivo* carcinogenicity.

General examples of the scientific and ethical necessity for public health of animal experiments can be given.

- For drugs, the problem of investigating reactions in pregnant women became essential after the thalidomide drama. Systematic evaluation of the action of drugs on the reproduction of at least two different species (sometimes including non-human primates) has probably avoided new dramas. If the efficacy of a potentially teratogenic drug is, nevertheless, of great therapeutic interest, its therapeutic use will be evaluated taking into account the ratio of benefit to risk, and the ability of patients to procreate.

- Chemical warfare is despicable, but we have seen recently that it can occur in especially cruel conflicts. We must therefore equip ourselves to fight this risk. In the case of nerve gases, extensive studies were and are still being done to find pharmacological antidotes. Taking into account the great difficulty of studying the nervous system, and the markers of intoxication (cholinesterases), only animal experiments can give relevant data in this field.

- Food additives are extensively used, and the human exposure is lifespan. This is why the international organizations (FAO – WHO, JECFA) have developed a successfully implemented policy of evaluation and re-evaluation of food additives by animal experiments. The outcome was that a large number of compounds were rejected or limited. In some cases, the mode of chemical synthesis was discovered to be responsible for the potential toxic action, so that it could be modified and the risk eliminated. Many compounds were discovered to be hepatotoxic, nephrotoxic, embryotoxic, carcinogenic, etc.; with all the toxic and ethical consequences of their use in man.

– Skin is our natural barrier and is, like the eyes, very exposed to aggressions by chemicals in occupational hazards, but also in domestic accidents, by drugs, cosmetics and such like. Investigations of irritation in animals have been widely criticized because of their eventual cruelty. Nevertheless, we must bear in mind that essential precautions for the handling, labelling, and use (cosmetics) of a large number of toxic compounds, with regular consequences for the safety of people, were established thanks to these investigations. It is obvious that limits must be defined for these assays, to avoid unacceptable pain to animals.

In every case, toxicologists must ensure animal welfare and avoid unnecessary pain. This assumption must be claimed not only for ethical considerations, but also to ensure the optimal scientific quality of the results of animal experiments; this is the basis of good laboratory practice.

4. Studies on *in vitro* or *ex vivo* models – cultured cells, perfused organs, cultured embryos, isolated skin – are extensively developed as models in toxicology for the future.

At present, these are presented as alternatives but are more like additional methods, especially useful for screening or for studies to elucidate the mechanism of action of the adverse effects of xenobiotics. In any case, we cannot consider that these models have the potency of an organism *in toto*, where all the interrelations between tissues and functions are respected. Furthermore, these methods have still to be validated, because all new methods proposed must be submitted to strict assessment before acceptance for regular use.

Under these conditions, the classic methods (animal experiments) should be in existence as long as it is not demonstrated that alternative methods provide an equivalent level of safety for man and his environment (EEC proposal).

We shall not spend too long on the use of additive methods here, because everybody knows that this question could be the topic of a full symposium. We shall just underline the fact that toxicologists must devote all their energies to promoting these methods, reducing the extent, cost and time taken for animal experiments.

5. Computer studies are not only the methodological end-point of statistical studies. Computer studies can help in simulations to compare well known chemical families of toxic xenobiotics with new compounds, on a structural and physico-chemical basis. The question here is not the extrapolation from

animals to man, but the extrapolation of comparable structural and physico-chemical properties to toxic effects. Obviously, this very rich approach cannot yet offer an adequate level for safety evaluation with regular consequences.

To conclude, in spite of all the questions concerning the ethical problem of animal welfare and the extrapolation from animal to man, this analysis indicated that, at present, animal experiments still appear to be the most suitable approach for safety evaluation from a scientific point of view as well as in a regular situation regarding public health.

Acknowledgements

to Mrs. M. Radionoff and Mrs. N. Thibault for their most appreciated contribution.

The necessity of animal testing for safety evaluation and medical progress in reproductive biology and toxicology

DIETHER NEUBERT
Institute for Toxicology and Embryopharmacology, Free University of Berlin, Berlin FRG

Introduction

The tragic experience gained from the thalidomide disaster in 1960–1962 has been the main reason for re-evaluating the requirements for 'safety assessment' in all areas of medical toxicology and for the development of new strategies by registration agencies all over the world. Until now, these strategies were based on extensive animal testing with all new drugs intended for use as medication and with all major environmental substances, in order to satisfy the high safety demands required by today's society.

On the other hand, accumulation of the basic medical knowledge on reproductive processes, predominantly gained through animal research, has made possible medical achievements such as embryo transfer and *in vitro* fertilization, hormone treatment during menopause, treatment of cancer of the reproductive organs, etc.

Aside from experimental designs using *in vivo* approaches, in recent decades *in vitro* techniques have become available and have been applied to several problems concerning development and reproduction. The applicability and limitation of these *in vivo* and *in vitro* methods in medical research in the field of reproductive and developmental biology and toxicity will be discussed.

Complexity of the reproductive and developmental sequence

Reproduction and development of the mammalian organism consist of thousands of extremely complex events and processes, many of which are only very poorly (or not at all) understood by us. It is a special characteristic of these biological events that they occur in a repeated sequence, spanning several generations. In this respect we are confronted with the most complex and significant biological phenomena nature has to offer (Fig. 1). Therefore, it is clear that to study this multiplicity of processes complex systems must be used.

The multiple events occurring during reproduction and development can

S. Garattini (ed.), The Importance of Animal Experimentation for Safety and Biomedical Research, 191–197.

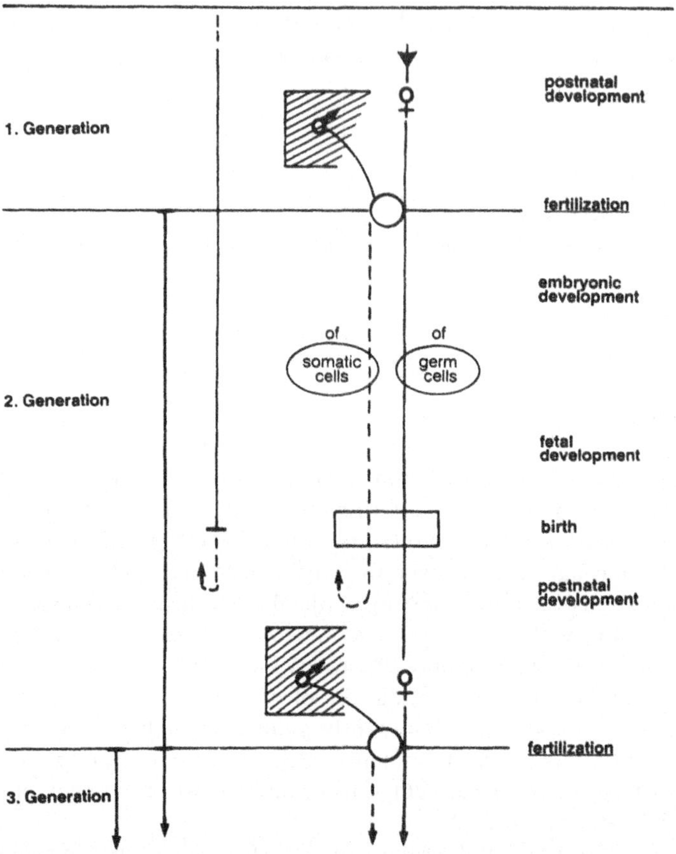

Fig. 1. Multigeneration sequence of reproduction and development. The sequence of events expands over several generations. Important is the extensive multiplicity of the adverse health effects that can be triggered during this prolonged period.

be disturbed at many levels, leading to a variety of abnormalities. Some of the major processes in the sequence mentioned are listed in Table 1.

Test systems used in reproductive and developmental biology and toxicology

Medical research in the field of reproduction and development has two basic goals:

- to understand normal processes and
- to understand abnormal development.

For such studies 'models' are used which, it is hoped, mimick the situations occurring in the human organism during these stages of development as closely as possible and from which certain common principles governing the devel-

Table 1. Processes in reproduction and development that may be effected by toxic substances

Male fertility	Placentation
Female fertility	Fetal development
Fertilization	Perinatal development
Preimplantation development	Parturition
Implantation	Lactation
Early postimplantation development	Postnatal development
Organogenesis	Etc.

opment of higher organisms up to the mammals, including man, can be identified. Such models can either be *in vivo* (such as the whole mammalian organism or 'simple' organisms studied during their development) or *in vitro*, i.e. parts of the reproductive sequence or of an organism growing in culture or even whole embryos cultured *in vitro* for short periods of time.

The test system chosen for studying a defined scientific problem depends strictly on the goal to be achieved. In principle it may be stated that the system should be chosen according to the problem (and not *vice versa*, as often done): if the problem is to seek a better understanding of the basic processes governing reproductive and developmental processes, a system as simple as possible may be a good choice, especially if comparative studies can be made.

The situation is entirely different if the goal of the studies is to exclude as far as possible all the different adverse effects that could interfere with the numerous processes during reproduction or development and possibly cause serious adverse health effects. This situation, which is typical in toxicology, will be difficult if knowledge already gathered on the substance in question is scant ('primary' stage testing). In a case like this it is of considerable advantage to have a system available as complex as possible, not too distant in biological complexity from the human organism. This, at out present level of scientific knowledge, will certainly be an intact mammalian organism.

In vivo systems used for risk assessment

In order to assess abnormal reproduction and development the whole sequence, extending over several generations, has to be evaluated. There are two ways to achieve this:

- either to perform a multigeneration study
- or to assess the events in separate experimental set-ups (Fig. 2). Such studies are the segments I, II and III.

A routine three-segment study, by today's standards necesssary for complete assessment of the possible reproductive toxicity of a substance, requires approximately 240 rats and 60 rabbits. Therefore, it is understandable that

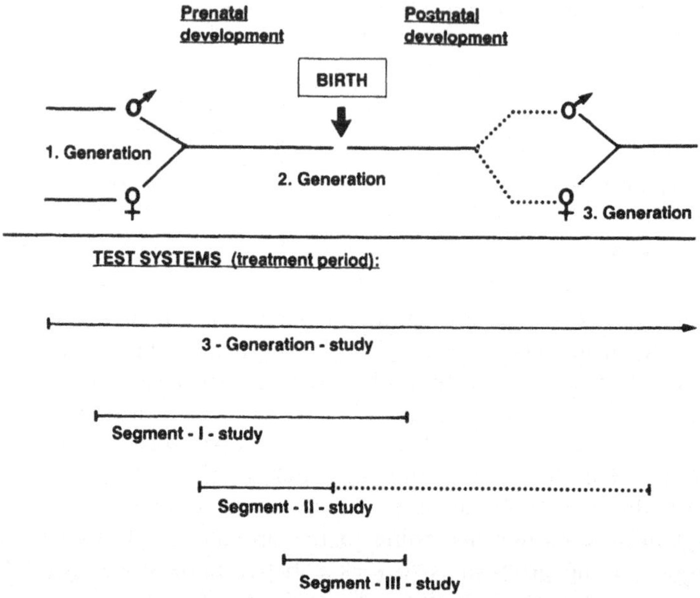

Fig. 2. In vivo test systems currently used for the assessment of reproductive or developmental toxicity. The many susceptible periods may be evaluated either by a multigeneration study, or by multiple test procedures (segments I to III) suitable for studying different and defined periods of development.

attempts have been made to reduce these numbers of animals and at the same time possibly reduce costs, time and manpower required.

In vitro systems available today

In the field of reproductive and developmental biology and toxicology numerous 'alternative' systems have been developed in recent years and several have been proposed (as yet without general acceptance) for the assessment of possible toxic risks. The term 'alternative' however, is unacceptable in medical research, it was 'invented' by laymen. In medical, as in other fields of research, there are only suitable and unsuitable methods for a certain purpose. If a method has been proved to be suitable it is, and has to be, used for this purpose. It cannot be an alternative. For this reason, *in vitro* methods, for example, are by no means new or alternatives. They have been used for decades (some of them longer than *in vivo* techniques) for certain purposes (e.g. isolated organs and tissues in pharmacological testing).

Therefore, the development and recognition of *in vitro* techniques was not stated up by recent attitudes towards reducing or replacing experimental animals. Claims in this direction are entirely wrong, and in fact no single

Table 2. Ranking scales of systems of varying biological complexity to be used in assessing toxic effects on reproduction and development

(1) Man	(2) Whole organism
Non-human primates	Whole embryo or fetus
Other mammals	Part of embryo or fetus
Chick	Differentiating tissue
Amphibia	Embryonic cells
Fish	Tissue cultures
'Lower organisms' such as	Cell cultures
Ciona, hydractinia, hydra,	Multi-enzyme complexes
etc.	Enzyme reactions
	Chemical reactions
	Computer 'simulations'?

technique has been developed by any special institution claiming to be scientifically active in this field. All prerequisites for using *in vitro* techniques in medical research have been developed in research institutions.

The systems available for research in reproductive or developmental toxicology may be ranked according to a number of criteria:

1. The phylogeny of the animals from which the tissues are derived (mammals vs. lower organisms);
2. The biological complexity of the material (whole organism vs. cell cultures).

The various organisms and the different biological complexities of systems used today as 'models' are set out in Table 2.

While in some of the organisms (e.g. amphibia) the whole period of development can be conveniently observed (it may drastically differ from that of mammals, though!), some other systems only allow evaluation of certain developmental processes, such as organogenesis (e.g. of the early limb in a limb bud culture of rodents).

Applicability and limitations of *in vitro* systems

Some of these *in vitro* systems are currently used extensively in many laboratories for 'secondary-stage testing', i.e. to supplement previously performed *in vivo* tests. For this purpose these systems have gained considerable importance and are now an integral part of the repertoire of systems available in a specialized laboratory.

It must be realized that none of the systems available until now is able to mimick the entire sequence of mammalian reproduction and development. Furthermore, most of the systems were designed to evaluate possible adverse effects on prenatal development, and very few (if any) were intended for investigating the other important parts of the above sequence.

The better systems available today use mammalian tissue. They are complex systems (such as whole-embryo culture or organ culture) and capable of showing differentiations (preferentially morphogenic differentiations, i.e. pattern formation). Nothing is known on the predictive value of very simple systems. Some of the 'advertised' systems (and in the USA even patented!) like the one using a simple hydra aggregation, are now known to be of no value at all.

A few examples of previously unrecognized adverse effects of a substance on prenatal development have been detected using the more complex *in vitro* techniques, such as the whole-embryo culture (Neubert *et al.*, 1986). These effects, initially seen *in vitro*, were subsequently confirmed *in vivo*, thus verifying the predictive value in these special cases.

None of these systems have been validated as yet for the complete replacement of *in vivo* tests during 'primary' stage testing. Primary stage testing means evaluation of a new substance for which very little (if any) previous information has been gathered.

Summary and possibilities for the future

The *in vitro* systems available so far do not permit an assessment of all the events occurring during mammalian reproduction and development. Such a goal can at present only be achieved through appropriate *in vivo* studies. The only field in which some progress has been made in recent years is prenatal development. Again, however, no system has been found (and no 'battery' of tests is known as yet) that would allow primary stage testing and provide a sufficient degree of safety, by present standards.

In reproductive toxicology *in vitro* techniques have largely enriched secondary-stage testing, i.e. the supplementation of *in vivo* studies. This should be considered an extremely important aspect, and laboratories using such techniques could not do without them anymore. Often the *in vitro* techniques offer better possibilities than *in vivo* ones, even those using large series of animals. Applications for such *in vitro* techniques include: to distinguish direct effects on the embryo from results of maternal toxicity, direct testing of metabolites, and especially the screening of series of derivatives with similar chemical structures in cases where the original substance *in vivo* induces a defined abnormality and where an appropriate *in vitro* system is available.

It should be borne in mind that all the *in vitro* systems (whole-embryo culture, organ cultures, micromass cultures, etc.), reasonably well suited for assessing prenatal toxic risk, still use mammalian or avian tissue and require the sacrifice of animals (although they may greatly help in reducing the number of animals required).

Very extensive work will be needed in the next decade to validate new *in vitro* techniques and it may become necessary to alter the safety demands of our population in this field, if a drastic reduction (or even abandon) of animal experiments is the final goal.

References

1. Merker H-J, Heger W, Sames K, Stürje H, Neubert D (1988) Embryotoxic effects of thalidomide-derivatives in the non-human primate callithrix jacchus – I. Effects of 3-(1,3-dihydro-1-oxo-2H-isoindol-2-yl)-2,6-dioxopiperidine (EM 12) on skeletal development. *Arch Toxicol* 61: 165–179
2. Neubert D, Barrach H-J, Merker H-J (1980) Drug-induced damage to the embryo or fetus (Molecular and multilateral aproach to prenatal toxicology). In: Grundman E (Ed) *Current topics in pathology*. Vol 69, Springer-Verlag, Berlin, Heidelberg, New York, pp 241–331
3. Neubert D (1982) The use of culture techniques in studies on prenatal toxicity. In: Papp G (Ed) *Pharmacology and therapeutics*. Vol 18, Pergamon Press, Oxford, pp 397–434
4. Neubert D (1985) Benefits and limits of model systems in developmental biology and toxicology (*in vitro* techniques). In: Marois M (Ed) *Prevention of physical and mental congenital defects, Part A: the scope of the problem*. Alan R Liss Inc, New York, pp 91–96
5. Neubert D (1985) Toxicity studies with cellular models of differentiation. *Xenobiotica* 15: 649–660
6. Neubert D, Blankenburg G, Lewandowski C, Klug S (1985) Misinterpretations of results and creation of 'artifacts' in studies on developmental toxicity using systems simpler than *in vivo* systems. In: Lash JW, Saxén L (Eds) *Developmental mechanisms, normal and abnormal, progress in clinical and biological research*. Vol 171, Alan R Liss Inc, New York pp 241–266
7. Neubert D, Chahoud I (1985) Significance of species and strain differences in pre- and perinatal toxicology. *Acta Histochem* 31: 23–35
8. Neubert D, Stahlmann R, Chahoud I, Bochert G (1985) Some aspects of prenatal toxicology. *Trends in Pharmacol Sci* 1985 (Fed Eur Soc Toxicol) Suppl: 1–6
9. Neubert D, Blankenburg G, Chahoud I, Franz G, Herken R, Kastner M, Klug S, Kröger J, Krowke R, Lewandowski C, Merker H-J, Schulz T (1986) Results of *in vivo* and *in vitro* studies for assessing prenatal toxicity. *Environ Health Perspect* 70: 89–103.
10. Neubert D (1986) Zur Vorhersehbarkeit von toxischen Risiken für den Menschen anhand von Ergebnissen aus *in vivo* und *in vitro* Versuchen. In: Burger EK, Grosdanoff P, Henschler D, Knaupp O, Schnieders B (Eds) *Aktuelle Probleme der Biomedizin*. Walter de Gruyter, Berlin, New York, pp 475–483
11. Neubert D, Bochert G, Platzek T, Chahoud I, Fisher B, Meister R (1987) Dose-response relationships in prenatal toxicity. *Congenit Anomalies* 27: 275–302
12. Neubert D, Chahoud I, Platzek T, Meister R (1987) Principles and problems in assessing prenatal toxicity. *Arch Toxicol* 60: 238–345
13. Neubert D (1988) Significance of pharmacokinetic variables in reproductive and developmental toxicity. *Xenobiotica* 18: 45–58
14. Neubert D, Heger W, Merker H-J, Sames K, Meister R (1988) Embryotoxic effects of thalidomide derivatives in the non-human primate callithrix jaccus – II. Elucidation of the susceptible period and of the variability of embryonic stages. *Arch Toxicol* 61: 180–191

The need for animal experimentation in studying the carcinogenic risk of substances

IRENE CHOUROULINKOV
Institute for Scientific Research on Cancer – CNRS, Laboratory of Experimental Carcinogenesis and Genetic Toxicology, Villejuif Cedex, France

Introduction

The influence of organisations on opinion against the use of animals for scientific experimentation has been so great these past few years that regulations have been developed introducing the control of and/or ban on the use of animals in experimental investigations. The essential argument of the associations for the protection of animals is the excesses of the experimentalists. It should be noted that excesses can be pointed out on both sides. Although some experimentalists exceed the acceptable limits defined by current ethics, others, truly conscious of the problem, have provided recommendations leading to an avoidance of superfluous experiments.

> 'Investigations in the animal have, as a primary objective, the assessment of risks of cancer to the human; complementary experiments should not be requested if the answer sought after can be obtained from observations in the human'.
>
> (Recommendation 3-2, ref. [1], p. 247)

The motivations of action for the majority of the members of the associations for the protection of animals are respectable and most frequently shared by research scientists. Nonetheless, members with excessive positions can be found amongst them. As an example, I would quote a paragraph from a letter I received after a visit to my laboratory by a group of members of an association protesting against the use of animals for experimental purposes.

> 'How is it that no one has tried, at least as far as we know, to experiment on delinquent humans, dissolute and political criminals, for example (there have been plenty of them these past few years)'. Mr. and Mrs. X.

The aims of my exposé are not to polemise on opinions, the positions and the regulations for the control of the use of animals in experimental investigations. We shall attempt to find, from historical data, the contribution made by tests on animals in the assessment of the risks of cancer to the human; to see to what degree the substitution tests (short-term trials) have fulfilled the hopes; to try to classify carcinogenic substances on mechanistic bases; and finally to suggest an experimental scheme for assessment of the

S. Garattini (ed.), The Importance of Animal Experimentation for Safety and Biomedical Research, 199–209.

carcinogenic risk of chemical products, thus allowing limitations to be placed on the systematic recourse to animals.

Assessment of the risk of cancer for the human: historical data

The first relationships between the exposure to a substance and the development of cancer in the human were based on clinical and epidemiological observations. These observations have placed blame on complex or pure substances as a causal agent in cancer and are at the basis of the notion of cancer development following professional exposure [2]. With few exceptions, these observations have been confirmed experimentally at least in animal species [3]. Out of 34 substances which are carcinogenic for the human (Table 1, group 1), for 20 substances the experimental data are largely sufficient to affirm that they are carcinogenic for animals; for 6 the data are not sufficient, but indicative enough; for 2 the studies were not adequate and finally for 6 there are no data.

Numerous *in vivo* investigations have been performed with various chemical products, the results of which have permitted a classification of 196 substances which cause cancer in animals and are probable carcinogens for the human (Table 1, groups 2A and 2B) [3].

Table 1. Overall assessment of the carcinogenicity of substances [3]

Groups	Substance number	Degree of evidence of carcinogenicity[a]		Classification
		Human	Animal	
1	34:20	S	S	carcinogenic substances for the human
	6	S	L	
	2	S	I	
	6	S	I	
2A	37	L	S	carcinogenic substances for the human
2B	159	I	S	possible carcinogenic substances for the human

[a] S = Sufficient evidence; L = light evidence; I = insufficient evidence or unknown (no study).

The conclusions drawn from these observations were, and still are, that chemical agents can have cancer risks for the human and that experiments on animals provide a means of detecting the carcinogenic capability, for assessing the risks to the human and for developing and recommending preventive measures. Taking as a basis the clinical and experimental observations, the participants in the Symposium on 'Potential Carcinogenic Hazards from Drugs' [1] made a number of recommendations, No. 4 of which states:

'The cancer risk should be assessed for any drug as an essential part of the general toxicological evaluation'.

This evaluation clearly concerned recourse to animal experimentation since, during the course of the same symposium, the principles of *in vivo* methodology were dealt with [4].

This recommendation, followed by others, as well as by the development of national and international rules and regulations on the control of all chemical products, implied an application effort which would be difficult to imagine. The number of chemical products on the market, the new substances proposed every year, and the substances in the environment was estimated to be several tens of thousands. The carcinogenic potential of such a number of substances could not be studied because of a lack of economic means and the very limited capabilities of existing laboratories equipped to carry out long-term *in vivo* investigations of carcinogens.

All these facts – the pressing problems of the control of chemical products, economic and ethical problems and the problem of application – imposed a search for methods and systems other than animals. The development of short-term tests of carcinogenic substances offered great hope that these problems could be solved, to the satisfaction of all involved. Thus, work on short-term tests of mutagenesis with a view to assessing the carcinogenic risk of substances was accelerated as of 1975. It is necessary to recall briefly why this occurred, what its contribution is and the place it has in the study of the carcinogenic risks of chemical products.

Short-term tests of carcinogenesis

The recommendation for short-term tests of mutagenesis for the assessment of carcinogenic risks was justified by economic, scientific and coordinational arguments.

The economic arguments are obvious: relatively low cost and time-savings. From a scientific point of view, carcinogenesis is assimilated to a phenomenon of mutation, DNA playing the role of principle target. Given the fact that DNA contains the genetic code, any lesion caused by an agent is likely to bring about mutation, and since DNA is the universal component of organisms, except RNA viruses, any agent which causes a lesion in the DNA of an organism is likely also to reach the DNA of human cells. The corollaries of these two postulates are the possibility of using a whole series of events as criteria of an effect between the attack on DNA and expression in the form of mutations, in an entire series of target organisms such as bacteria, yeasts, cells in culture, *Drosophila*, mammals and plants. Finally, the main justification came from the demonstration that the majority of known carcinogens are mutagenic in bacteria. The reverse should also be true [5].

Investigations using short-term tests of mutagenesis and the data accumulated over a dozen years are so considerable that it would be pretentious and dangerous to attempt to summarise them. It suffices to consult the scientific journals and the results obtained within the context of the IPCS (International program for Chemical Safety), WHO [6, 7], and NTP (National Toxicology Program) NIEHS, USA programmes.

I shall simply state that during the course of the 'EPA Workshop on Relationships between Short-term Test Information and Carcinogenicity' (Williamsburg, Virginia, USA, January 20–23, 1987), it was reported that the sensitivity or specificity of the tests varied as a function of the laboratory systems, the combination of tests, etc.... The final conclusion was:

> 'No one test system or combination of test systems will accurately identify the universe of carcinogens or non-carcinogens'. (A. Auletta)

In effect, the short-term tests single out four groups of substances: [1] mutagenic and carcinogenic substances, [2] non-mutagenic but carcinogenic substances, [3] mutagenic but non-carcinogenic substances, and [4] non-mutagenic and non-carcinogenic substances (Table 2).

The explanations put forth for the substances in group 3e, the false negatives in assays of carcinogenesis, are that the specificity of the organ, the line or species, the inadequate route of administration, the weak sensitivity of *in vivo* trials or the incorrect performance of the trials, may provide negative results. However, there is also the question of false positives in tests of mutagenesis. Thus, it is supposed that lesions in the DNA are repaired *in vivo*, or that the genotoxic effects are not linked to the induction of tumours, or finally that the *in vitro* and *in vivo* physiological conditions were not identical – detoxification, for example.

These justifications are plausible. Nonetheless, they are not sufficient to explain why 3-methyl-4-nitroquinoline-N-oxide (3M-4NQO), which is as mutagenic as 4-nitroquinoline-N-oxide (4NQO) is not carcinogenic. The same question arises for 1-naphthylamine and 4-acetylaminofluorene, which have been shown to be mutagenic in a number of tests [8]. The author considers that, lacking a rational explanation, other long-term tests of carcinogenicity are needed. Personally I would ask the following question: is the genotoxic effect sufficient for the development of a tumour *in vivo*? This question is the logical follow-up to one of the explanations that the genotoxic effects

Table 2. Groups of substances as a function of short and long-term tests and mode of action. Level of action and possible risk

Groups	Carcinogen	Mutagen	Mode of action	Carcinogenesis in two phases	Level of action	Possible risk
Gr.1	+	+	genotoxic epigenetic	initiator promotor	DNA membrane cytoplasm tissue	High
Gr.2	+		epigenetic	promotor		Low
Gr.3		+	genotoxic	initiator	DNA	Low
Gr.4		–	–	–		No risk

are probably not linked to the induction of tumours *in vivo*. Moreover, this explanation implicitly admits the existence of another mechanism. In effect, the substances in group 2 are carcinogenic without being mutagenic. In the discussion of the results of short-term tests with diethylhexylphthalate, diethylstilboestrol, phenobarbital and benzene, the possibility of the existence of non-genotoxic carcinogens (epigenetic agents) was brought up [9]. TPA (12-O-tetradecanoyl-phorbol-13-acetate) is a non-genotoxic carcinogen [10, 11].

These explanations and the proof that non-genotoxic substances may induce tumours lead to the conclusion that the genotoxic effect is not necessary.

Therefore, how can the carcinogenic action of genotoxic substances such as benzo(a)pyrene (BaP) and 7,12-dimethyl-benz(a)anthracene (CMBA) be explained? The explanations proposed were that part of the substance acted as an initiator and another part as promotor, or that some metabolites were initiators and others promotors. Unfortunately, none of these arguments explains the carcinogenic action of a high dose. The rapid disappearance of the substance cannot play the role of promotor. It is necessary to admit and prove that these substances have a double genotoxic and epigenetic action. The effects of the epigenetic action are reversible, and this explains why low doses are only initiating agents. Conversely, high doses create irreversible tissue and probably cellular lesions.

Mechanistic classification of chemical carcinogens

The discussion of the relationship between the short-term tests and the carcinogenicity of the substances led to a classification of these substances in four groups: double-action carcinogens (genotoxic and epigenetic) (group 1), epigenetic carcinogens (non-genotoxic) (group 2), genotoxic carcinogens (mutagens) (group 3) and non-carcinogens (group 4) (Table 2) [12]. In any case, this classification was also based on experimental results.

During the course of a study on the relation and structure of three naphthofurans: 2-nitro-7-methoxy-naphtho(2-1b)furan (A), 2-nitro-naphtho(2-1b)furan (C) and 7-methoxy-naphtho(2-1b)furan (E), recourse was successively to tests of mutagenesis, short and long-term cutaneous tests in the mouse. The short-term cutaneous tests, the sebaceous gland and epidermal hyperplasia tests were predictive of a potential carcinogenic risk but especially of a promoting potential or action by the epigenetic route [13] (Table 3).

Looking at the results of the mutagenesis and short-term cutaneous tests we predicted for substance A a predominant initiator (genotoxic) potential, for C a promotor (epigenetic) potential and for E no action. These predictions were confirmed in the long-term cutaneous test of carcinogenicity (Table 3) [12, 14–16]. However, substance E was found to be highly carcinogenic, more carcinogenic than TPA, which is much more active in the hyperplasia test and is not mutagenic. Thus, the carcinogenic activity of substance C could not be explained exclusively by an epigenetic mechanism. In fact, substance

Table 3. Study of the mutagenic and carcinogenic activity of three nitronaphthofurans [12, 14, 15]

Substance	Mutagenic activity[a]	Activity in short-term cutaneous T[b]	Activity in long-term cutaneous T[c]		
			Init.	Prom.	Carc.
2-Nitro-7-methoxy-naphtho(2-1b)furan (A)	++++	++	+++++	++	+
2-Nitro-*naphtho*-(2-1b)furan (C)	++	++++	+	++++	+++
7 methoxy-naphtho-(2-1b)furan (E)	–	+	–	+	–
TPA[d] [13]	–	+++++	–	+++++	–

[a] Results of eight *in vitro* and *in vivo* tests (T) of mutagenesis.
[b] Sebaceous gland and epidermal hyperplasia tests.
[c] (Init)iator – the product – one application followed by treatment with TPA;
(Prom)otor – repeated applications on mice pre-treated with BaP;
(Carc)inogen – the product alone – repeated applications.
[d] TPA – 12-O-tetradecanoyl-phorbol-13-acetate.

C was found to be mutagenic. It is less active than A, but this activity is sufficient to be taken into consideration, which permits substance C to be classified in group 1, with double genotoxic and epigenetic action. Substance E is in group 4, while TPA is in group 2 (epigenetic) according to Table 2.

During investigations of the role of solvents in cutaneous carcinogenesis, it was found that the activity of BaP, DMBA and TPA in short-term cutaneous tests was prevented when arachis oil was used as a solvent. In the long-term cutaneous test, tumour development was also inhibited when BaP and DMBA were in solution in arachis oil. The promoting action of TPA on mice initiated with DMBA was equally inhibited. However BaP binding to the DNA of epidermal cells was not blocked (Table 4) [17]. This indicates that arachis oil prevents the epigenetic action at the level of epidermal cells only, since it did not block sarcomatogenic action in the rat, thus confirming the classification of BaP and DMBA in group 1.

Dexamethasone (DM) is an anti-inflammatory and anti-promoting agent [19]. It was thought possible to verify whether the epigenetic effect, expressed in the form of hyperplasia or transformed colonies (system of Syrian Hamster embryo cells (SHE)) was induced by carcinogens. The development of hyperplasia was in fact prevented when the treatments with BaP and DMBA (Table 4) and TPA (not reported) were followed 1 hour later by an application of DM. Likewise, the formation of transformed colonies on SHE cells treated with BaP was inhibited, without inhibition of its binding to cellular macromolecules (Chouroulinkov *et al.*, unpublished results). These results indicate that epidermal hyperplasia and the formation of transformed colonies on SHE cells are criteria of epigenetic effects, and by using inhibitors with molecular

Table 4. Action of BaP, DMBA, 4NQO and 3M-4NQO as a function of the test (T) and the solvent and the association with dexamethasone

	BaP			DMBA		4NQO	3M-4NQO
	A[a]	P.O.[a]	DM	A	P.O.	A	A
Short-term cutaneous T of carcinogenesis	+++	–	–	+++	–	++	–
Long-term cutaneous T of carcinogenesis	+++	–	n.p.	+++	–	++ [18]	– [18]
SHE cells in culture (transformed)	++	n.a.	–	n.p.	n.p.	n.p.	n.p.
DNA binding	++	++	++	n.p.	n.p.	n.p.	n.p.

[a] A = acetone; P.O. = arachis oil; DM = dexamethasone; n.a. = not adequate; n.p. = not performed.

analysis the genotoxic and epigenetic action can be identified.

According to this logic, the 4NQO and 3-4NQO pair were considered, using the hypothesis that 4NQO has double action (group 1), while 3M-4NQO is only genotoxic (group 3), and this genotoxic action is not sufficient to induce tumours. In short-term cutaneous tests, 4NQO was positive, while 3M-4NQO was negative (Table 4) (Chouroulinkov *et al.*, unpublished). The hypothesis was confirmed; 4NQO has double action (group 1) and 3M-4NQO is only genotoxic (group 3). It remains necessary to verify whether dexamethasone prevents the hyperplasia effect of 4NQO without affecting its interaction with cellular DNA.

Application

The mechanistic classification of carcinogenic agents (Table 2) confirmed in short-term cutaneous tests and partially also on the system of SHE cells, allows the role of each substance in the operative system to be forecast based on the concept of dual-phase carcinogenesis – initiation/promotion. The substances in group 1, at low doses, can play the role of initiator, those in group 2 the role of promotors and finally, the substances in group 4 should play the role of initiators. For these latter substances, there are currently no adequate data to really substantiate their role as initiator. Experiments with metabolites of BaP have shown an initiator effect on the skin of mice, but the same metabolites injected subcutaneously in the rat had no sarcomatogenic action, contrary to BaP [20]. In fact, these metabolites form adducts with epidermal and conjunctival cellular DNA [21]. These results indicate that there are genotoxic and non-carcinogenic substances.

Depending on the mode of action and the experimental data, the level of action of the various groups of substances can be situated. As regards the skin, there is a level of epidermal cells: DNA as target (genotoxic effect), the membrane and the cytoplasm (epigenetic effect) and a level of conjunctival tissue (inflammatory reaction) (Table 2). Cells in culture can detect genotoxic (binding to DNA, mutation) and epigenetic (morphological, biological and biochemical criteria) effects.

Pragmatically speaking, the diagram below seems to provide the solution to the problems of detection and assessment of the carcinogenic potential of substances and thus limits, but does not eliminate, recourse to the use of animals.

Diagram of investigation of the carcinogenic potential of substances

Mutagenesis tests

Positive (Genotoxic)			Negative (Non-genotoxic)

- Short-term cutaneous tests (mouse)
- Test of cellular transformation in culture

Positive (Group 1)	Negative (Group 3)	Positive (Group 2)	Negative (Group 4)

This diagram appears simple and attractive, but like any biological test, the short-term cutaneous tests have limits. They can be used for the majority of organo-soluble and more or less organo-specific substances. The hepatocarcinogens such as 2-AAF have no effect on the skin of the mouse. To overcome this disadvantage, systems of cell transformation in culture may play the role of complementary test. Currently, two cellular systems are used: Balb/3T3 cells and Syrian hamster embryo cells [23]. However other models which better represent the various organs must be developed because the other disadvantage of short term tests on skin and cells in culture is that long-term effects cannot be predicted.

The results

The results with the naphthofurans (Table 3) revealed that substance A is mildly carcinogenic for the skin and substance C is highly carcinogenic. However, systematic anatomo-pathological examination of the animals showed that substance A had caused tumour development in the oesophagus and the fore-stomach in 60% of the treated mice. Conversely, the mice treated with substance C revealed no tumour in the long term which could be imputed to the treatment. It appears that metabolites or substance A itself act in the long term through an epigenetic route. The tumours covered large areas and at their onset a bipolar proliferation of the basal layer was noted, as if the basal membrane did not exist or did not fulfill its physiological role of preventing deep proliferation of epithelial cells. This is not an isolated example. It is all too well known from investigations or oral carcinogenesis that not only the digestive tract is involved.

These facts indicate that recourse to animals is necessary when the various *in vivo* events which lead to tumour development have not been understood. Indeed, these events are multiple and complex. I. Penn [24] reported that the Cincinnati Transplant Registry noted 2063 tumours between 1968 and 1984 out of 1934 patients having a transplanted organ. The author points out multiple tumours in 346 out of 689 cases (44%) and a very short latency time: 30 survivors (of 418) 10 years after renal transplant, 14 (46%) of whom had tumours. In order to prevent rejection of the transplant, the patients had received immunosuppressive treatments involving agents which acted on the immune system by the epigenetic route, and agents which were genotoxic, mutagenic, even carcinogenic, the latter often being used in chemotherapy for cancer. It is now known that the sequential or simultaneous association of group 1 or group 3 agents with group 2 agents has sinergistic effects. A single low dose of BaP does not induce tumours. Associated with TPA, however, which is itself mildly carcinogenic at the adopted dose and frequency of application, it induced a startling number of tumours on the skin of the mouse. It should be noted that no experimental investigations have been carried out on the carcinogenic effect of associations of immunodepressors and genotoxic substances used to treat patients having received organ transplants. Nonetheless, the problem is of consequence and must not be ignored.

Benefitting from this information, it can be stated that the substances of group 1 and associations between groups 1 and 2 or groups 3 and 2 have a high cancer risk (Table 2). Taken separately, groups 2 and 3 have a relatively low risk. It all depends on the exposure conditions: single or multiple doses, treatment period, etc. The prediction of risks is important and the assessment in animals, *in vivo*, is necessary when chemical products which cannot be isolated from the general or professional environment, as well as medicaments, are involved. In the latter case, the decision to use the substance in therapy depends on the risk/benefit ratio. This ratio will be better assessed using results from animals than if based on predicted results of short-term tests. It is true that the extrapolation of animal findings to the human is not always easy, but the physiological conditions and measurements will be closer to those in man.

Conclusions

As a sort of conclusion, I would like to point out that my attitude during the course of my career has been to try to understand and to apply the knowledge acquired by attempting to reduce recourse to the use of animals for experiments on carcinogenesis. I believe this attitude is reflected in my exposé.

I am convinced that we have arrived at a degree of progress in knowledge, permitting some predictive conclusions regarding carcinogenesis based on data provided by short-term tests to be made. However, this progress does not yet warrant the neglecting of *in vivo* investigations for the study of the mechanisms of carcinogenesis and the assessment of cancer risks. The clearly carcinogenic agents (group 1) have already been catalogued or are easy to catalogue. There remain the agents having a mysterious, so-called epigenetic action, the mechanisms of which are closely linked to the development and control of the physiological equilibrium of the higher beings such as man. In terms of molecular biology, the epigenetic mechanisms are implicated in the control of genetic expression. In terms of carcinogenesis, this control is limited to the expression of genes linked to the division and secondary differentiations of various types of cells making up the organism. Thus, the epigenetic systems and control mechanisms in a complex organism cannot be entirely elucidated using cellular models in culture, which have only to do with cellular biology. The *in vivo* reference is absolutely indispensable for investigation of these mechanisms and for assessment of cancer risks. There remains the decision concerning the choice of species – the human or the rodent. Personally, I recommend the rodent.

References

1. Potential Carcinogenic Hazards from Drugs. Evaluation of Risks (1967) R Truhaut (Ed) U.I.C.C. Monogr. Series, Vol. 7, Springer-Verlag, Berlin, Heidelberg, N. York
2. Shimkin MB, Triolo VA (1969) History of chemical carcinogenesis: some prospective remarks. *Prog Exp Tumor Res* Vol. 11: 1–20, Karger, Basel, N. York
3. IARC (1987) Monographs on the evaluation of carcinogenic risks to humans. Supplement 7, Lyon
4. Berenblum I (1967) Principles of methodology relating to the potential carcinogenicity of medical drugs. R Truhaut (Ed) *Carcinogenic Potential Hazard from Drugs*, Springer-Verlag, Berlin, Heidelberg, N. York, 28–32
5. McCann J, Ames BN (1976) Detection of carcinogens as mutagens in the Salmonella/microsome test: assay of 300 chemicals, Part II. *Proc Natl Acad Sci* USA, 73: 950–954
6. Evaluation of short-term tests for carcinogens (1980) FJ de Serres, J Ashby (Eds), *Progress Mut Res*, Vol 1, Elsevier/North Holland
7. Evaluation of short-term tests for carcinogens (1985) J Ashby, FJ de Serres, M Draper, M Ishidate Jr, BH Margolin, GB Matter, MD Shelby (Eds): *Progress Mut Res* Vol 5, Elsevier Sci. Publishers, Amsterdam
8. Ashby J (1980) Overview of study and test chemical activities. In: FJ de Serres, J Ashby (Eds) *Evaluation of short-term tests for carcinogens*, 112–172, Elsevier/North Holland
9. Ashby J, de Serres FJ, Draper M, *et al.* (1985) Overview and conclusions of the IPCS collaborative study on *in vitro* assay systems. In: J Ashby *et al.* (Ed) *Evaluation of short-term tests for carcinogens*, 117–174, Elsevier, Amsterdam
10. Chouroulinkov I, Lazar P (1974) Action cancérogène et cocancérigène du 12-O-tétradécanoyl-phorbol-13-acétate (TPA), sur la peau de souris. *CR Acad Sci* Paris, 278D: 3027–3030
11. Astrup EG, Iversen OH (1983) The tumorigenic and carcinogenic effect of 12-O-tetradecanoyl-phorbol-13-acetate when applied to the skin of BALB/cA and hairless mice. *Acta Pathol Microbiol Scand* Sect A, 91–103
12. Chouroulinkov I (1968) Initiation, promotion: working concept, biological and toxicological interpretation of carcinogenesis. In: HO Iversen (Ed) *Theories of Carcinogenesis*, 191–201, Hemisphere Publ. Co., Washington
13. Lazar P, Chouroulinkov I (1974) Validity of the sebaceous glands test and the hyperplasia

test for the prediction of the carcinogenicity of cigarette smoke condensates and fractions. In: E Karbe, F Park (Eds) *Experimental Lung Cancer*, 383–391, Springer-Verlag, Berlin, Heidelberg, N. York

14. Venegas W, Sala M, Buisson JP, Royer R, Chouroulinkov I (1984) Relationship between the chemical structure and the mutagenic and carcinogenic potentials of five naphthofurans. *Cancer Res*, 33, 1969–1975
15. Venegas W, Lasne C, Lowy R, Buisson J-P, Chouroulinkov I (1985) Naphthofurans induced chromosomal aberrations detected in metaphase, anaphase and telophase V79 Chinese hamster cells. *Mutation Res*, 157: 53–62
16. Lasne C, Venegas W, Royer R, Chouroulinkov I (1987) Initiating, promoting and carcinogenic activities of three naphthofurans in mouse skin long term test. *Jpn J Cancer Res* (Ganne), 78: 565–570
17. Lasne C, Nguyen-Ba G, Chouroulinkov I (1988) Inhibition of chemical skin carcinogenesis in mice by arachis oil in an excipient. *Proc Amer Assoc Cancer Res*, Vol. 29: 163
18. Chemistry and biological actions of 4-nitroquinoline-1-Oxide (1971) E Endo, T Ono, T Sugimura (Eds), 32–52, Springer-Verlag, Berlin, Heidelberg, N. York
19. Belman S, Troll W (1972) The inhibition of croton oil-promoted mouse skin tumorigenesis by steroid hormones. *Cancer Research*, 32: 450–454
20. Chouroulinkov I, Gentil A, Tierney B, Grover PL, Sims P (1979) Biological activities of di-hydrodiols derived from two polycyclic hydrocarbons in rodent test systems. *Br J Cancer*, 39: 376–382
21. Rojas M, Baer-Dubowska W, Alexandrov K (1986) Comparison of benzo(a)pyrene-DNA adduct levels in mouse and rat epidermis and dermis. *Cancer Lett*, 30: 35–39
22. Kakunaga I (1973) A quantitative system for assay of malignant transformation by chemical carcinogens using a clone derived from BALB/3T3. *Int J Cancer*, 12: 463–473
23. DiPaolo JA (1980) Quantitative in vitro transformation of Syrian golden hamster embryo cells with the use of frozen stored cells. *J Natl Cancer Inst*, 64: 1485–1489
24. Penn I (1987) The consequences of immunodepression. In: A Berlin, J Dean, MH Draper, EMB Smith, F Spreafico (Eds) *Immunotoxicology*, 69–82, Martinus Nijhoff Publishers, Dordrecht (Netherlands)

THE FUTURE OF ANIMAL RESEARCH

Transgenic animals for human diseases and gene therapy

MARA ROSSINI, ELISABETTA DI MARTINO and GIULIANO BENSI
Sclavo Research Centre, Molecular Biology Labs, Siena, Italy

Introduction

The stable transfer of genetic information into the mouse germ line has become a well-established and powerful experimental technique [1–4].

Gene transfer is obtained by microinjecting a solution of DNA into one of the pronuclei of a fertilized egg (one cell embryo) and its subsequent implantation into the oviduct of a pseudopregnant female mouse. About 20-30% of the mice born acquire the injected DNA (transgenic mice) which is generally integrated as head-to-tail tandem array in a single (random) site. The result is a line of mice which inherits and transmits to its progeny the acquired 'transgene' that is usually expressed properly.

Transgenic mice provide a unique experimental model to explore the complex molecular biological effects of a gene in a living animal. Using this new technique it is possible to study the molecular basis of tissue-specific and stage-specific gene expression during development, and the phenotype effects of altered gene expression.

By fusing heterologous promoters with native structural gene it is possible, in transgenic animals, to modulate the amount of a gene product, to express it prematurely during development or to redirect its expression to cells that do not normally transcribe the gene. In this way, several pathological states reproducing human diseases have been obtained. They provide an experimental model of great value both for studies on the molecular mechanism of the disease and for pharmacological and therapeutic studies.

Alternatively, the introduction of foreign genes into mutant strains manifesting a pathological state has been used to cure the naturally occurring disorder (gene therapy).

Consequences of transgene expression

The ability to amplify the expression of a gene product or to target it to heterologous cell types by using strong promoters and tissue-specific elements

S. Garattini (ed.), The Importance of Animal Experimentation for Safety and Biomedical Research, 213–221.

has many potential applications for dissecting aspects of complex systems not accessible to *in vitro* analysis.

Alteration in growth control

In mammals, normal growth is under complex genetic and hormonal regulation. Central to this control is the interaction of the neuropeptides such as somatostatin and growth hormone releasing factor (GRF) with somatotroph cells thereby modulating the synthesis of growth hormone (GH). The binding of GH to receptors in the liver stimulates the production of insulin-like growth factor-1 (IGF-1) which in turn is thought to be a general stimulus for cell proliferation.

Transgenic mice have been produced with genes coding for GH, somatostatin and GRF fused to the metallothionein (MT) promoter to allow elevated and prolonged production of these peptides [5–9]. The most obvious effect of elevated production of GH or GRF in transgenic mice is stimulation of growth starting at about 3 weeks of age and reaching a plateau at about 12 weeks, when the mice are twice their normal size [5–7].

A number of other physiological processes are also affected in transgenic mice for GH. The chronic and ectopic production of GH feedback inhibits endogenous GH synthesis, leading to a marked reduction of the size of the pituitary glands which histologically resemble those of mice with a genetic deficiency in GH production (lit/lit mice) [10]. GH also impinges on sexual differentiation of the liver. The mRNA for the major urinary protein (MUP), which is normally the most abundant mRNA in the liver of males, is suppressed to very low levels in transgenic mice expressing GH chronically [11]. Ectopic GH production prevents fertility in females (not in males) and the animals show signs of premature aging.

The abnormal expression of human GRF in transgenic mice resulted in accelerated growth rates, as well as in measurable amounts of hGRF and increased levels of mouse GH in plasma. The pituitary glands of these animals were markedly hyperplastic. Thus, GRF acts as a specific growth factor for somatotroph cells as well as a regulator of GH gene expression and secretion. The animals were analogous to humans with a growth disorder associated with elevated serum GH pituitary hyperplasia, and sometimes a GRF-secreting tumor of the pancreas or bronchus [12].

The ectopic production of somatostatin in transgenic mice has no effect on growth; however, in this case processing of the precursor polypeptide was abnormal in most tissues [8].

Growth disorder in transgenic mice has also been achieved by introduction of a foreign dehydrofolate reductase (DHFR) gene [13]. The transgenic animals showed retarded growth and reduced fertility, pigmentation changes and skeletal defects. These defects are transmitted as dominant traits in several transgenic lines and are probably due to alteration in folate metabolism.

A variety of endocrine cells develop within the anterior pituitary specialized in the synthesis and secretion of different hormones such as GH, prolactin (PRL), gonadotropins (FSH and LH), corticotropin (ATCH) and thyrotropin (TSH). The precise lineal relationships among all these endocrine cells is not yet established. However there is some evidence that GH-synthesizing cells (somatotropes) and PRL-synthesizing cells (lactotropes) may derive from a common precursor that synthesizes both gene products [14].

Recently, a region of 310 base pairs located at the 5′ of the rat growth hormone gene was defined as being necessary and sufficient to direct the expression of hybrid genes to GH-expressing cell types. These GH 5′ sequences were used to direct the expression of diphtheria toxin to GH-expressing cells in the anterior pituitary gland of transgenic mice [15].

Such animals have impaired growth, reproductive difficulties and neurological symptoms. Ablation of GH-expressing cells during development resulted in the birth of normal pups, suggesting that GH is not required during embryogenesis. By 7 weeks of age however the transgenic pups were one third to half the size of their normal littermates. Serum GH was undetectable and plasma IGF-1 levels were reduced eight-fold in comparison to control animals, indicating GH-dependence of IGF-1 expression. The pituitaries were about a quarter the size of normal controls, GH-synthesizing cells were virtually non-existent and PRL-synthesizing cells were also reduced in number although not to the same extent as in GH-synthesizing cells, suggesting there may be more than one lineage pathway for their development. This model of genetic ablation of specific cell types illustrates the utility of this experimental animal system for understanding cell lineage of a particular cell type in morphogenesis. It also serves as a model of a hormone-deficient animal.

Oncogenesis

To study the properties and consequences of oncogene expression in transgenic mice, natural and recombinant oncogenes have been used (Table 1). A natural oncogene is defined as one in which the coding sequence is under the control of regulatory sequences of the gene itself. In contrast, a recombinant oncogene is one in which the structural transforming gene is fused to heterologous regulatory sequences in order to direct the expression to specific tissues.

The most extensively studied transforming gene in transgenic mice is the gene coding for the SV40 large T antigen. In transgenic mice the expression of SV40 early gene (coding for large and small T antigen) directed by its own promoter/enhancer sequences produces choroid plexus papillomas or carcinomas [16]. A detailed analysis has shown that the SV40 enhancer sequences (72 bp repeat region) were sufficient to target the expression in choroid plexus and only the expression of large T antigen is required to induce tumors [17]. When the enhancer sequences of SV40 early gene were deleted and the expression of large T antigen was driven by the metallothionein promoter, the transgenic animals showed different pathological states including dismyelinating peripheral neuropathy, hepatocellular carcinomas or islet cell

Table 1. Tumors induced in transgenic mice

Oncogene	Regulatory region promoter/enhancer	Phenotype	Reference
SV40 early region (large T Ag)	SV40 early promoter	Choroid plexus papillomas	[16] [17] [18]
SV40 early region (large T Ag)	Rat Elastase	Pancreatic acinar cell tumors	[19]
SV40 early region (large T Ag)	Rat Insulin	Insulinomas	[20]
SV40 early region (large T Ag)	SV40 enhancer + mouse MT promoter	Peripheral neuropathy, multifocal tumors, hepatomas, islet cell adenoma	[21]
SV40 early region (large T Ag)	Adenovirus E1	Glioblastomas	[22]
SV40 early region (large T Ag)	α-A-crystalline	Lens tumors	[23]
c-myc	c-myc	No effects	[24]
c-myc	Mouse MT	No effects	[24]
c-myc	MMTV-LTR	Mammary tumors	[25]
c-myc	Mouse Ig enhancer	B-cell lymphomas	[24]
c-myc	SV40 early region	Occasional tumors	[24]
Ha-ras	Rat elastase	Fetal exocrine pancreatic tumors	[26]
Ha-ras	MMTV-LTR	Mammary and salivary gland tumors	[27]
Ha-ras	WAP promoter	Mammary tumors	[28]
Polyoma Middle T Ag	Polyoma early region (ori-)	Hemangiomas	[29]
Bovine papilloma Virus I	Bovine Papilloma Virus I	Skin tumors	[30]
JC and BK viruses	JC and BK viruses	Kidney tumors	[31]
tat	HTLV-I/LTR	Mesenchymal tumors	[32]

MMTV = mouse mammary tumor virus; LTR = Long terminal repeat; WAP = whey acidic protein; HTLV-I = human T-lymphotropic virus type 1; MT = metallothionein; E1 = Early region 1.

adenomas of the pancreas [21]. The peripheral neuropathy was similar to Dejerine-Sottas neuropathy in man [33] and the peripheral nerve lesion to the trembler mouse (shiverer) mutants [34].

Pancreatic adenomas and insulinomas have been produced in transgenic mice with promoter/enhancer elements from the elastase I and insulin genes respectively, fused to SV40 T antigen gene [19,20].

On the other hand, transgenic mice bearing the *tat* gene of human T-lymphotropic virus type I under the control of its own long terminal repeat (LTR) were affected by multiple tumors of the sheaths of peripheral nerves [32] resembling von Recklinghausen's multiple neurofibromatosis in man [35].

By producing transgenic mice for c-myc gene fused to immunoglobin heavy chain enhancer (Eμ), Adams *et al.* [24] showed that the c-myc is a potent inducer of lymphomas. Mice bearing this transgene frequently had leukemia with massively enlarged lymph nodes, splenomegaly and enlarged thymus. The natural c-myc gene with its 5′ flanking sequences or the truncated form lacking the non-coding first intron were unable to induce tumors in transgenic mice.

The promoter/enhancer sequences from the mouse mammary tumor virus (MMTV) have been fused to either c-myc [25] or v-Ha-ras gene [27]. The transgenic mice obtained with these recombinant oncogenes developed neoplasm in the mammary gland. Mice bearing the c-myc oncogene develop tumors after a long latency suggesting that a secondary event must occur before the tumor can form. The second noteworthy characteristic is that the expression of the transgene in a different tissue (for example, salivary gland) does not necessarily lead to tumor formation.

The MMTV/v-Ha-ras transgenic mice present diffuse hyperplasia of the Harderian gland, or focal malignant neoplasm of mammary or salivary gland and lymphoid tissue. The Harderian gland hyperplasia seems to need only the action of the v-Ha-ras oncogene, whereas focal malignancies probably require additional somatic events.

The two strains of transgenic mice (MMTV/c-myc and MMTV/v-Ha-ras) have been crossed to produce hybrid mice in which the action of the two oncogenes causes a dramatic and synergistic acceleration of oncogenesis [27].

Specific diseases

Since the establishment of the transgenic mice technique several attempts have been made to produce an animal model for human insulin-dependent diabetes mellitus (IDMM). This pathology in humans is thought to result from both genetic and epigenetic components. The genetic component consists of at least one gene in the major histocompatibility complex (MHC) that contributes to susceptibility to the disease. For the disease to develop, some epigenetic triggering events must also occur. Experimentally these triggering events can be mimicked by either pharmacological or infectious agents, including several viruses.

Transgenic mice have been produced with Class II MHC A^d_α–A^d_β [36] or E^d_α–E^b_β [37], Interferon (IFN) γ [36] and Class I MHC H-2K^b [38] genes whose ectopic expression in pancreatic beta cells were directed by the regulatory region of the insulin gene. In all cases IDDM developed as a result of depletion of pancreatic beta cells. In the case of IFN γ, cell depletion was associated with an inflammatory process. None of these models created a pathology phenocopy of what is thought to be the general progression of the disease in human diabetes, although each recapitulated part of the damage noted. No lymphocytic infiltration was observed in histological sections of the pancreas from transgenic mice, indicating that islet destruction was not immunomediated and therefore that aberrant MCH expression does not directly induce autoimmunity, even though it is sufficient *per se* to cause beta cell destruction.

Table 2. Models of human pathology in transgenic mice

Construct	Pathological state	Reference
Rabbit β-globin	Thalassemia	[39]
mMT-1/rGH	Increased somatic growth	[6]
mMT-1/hGHRF	Increased somatic growth	[7]
mMT-1/Transthyretin	Amyloidosis	[40]
HPRT ES cells	Lesh-Nyhan syndrome	[41]
mMT-1/c-fos	Abnormal long bone development	[42]
rGH/DT	Dwarfism	[15]
antisense MBP	Trembler mouse (shiverer)	[43]
hIns/A^d_α,A^d_β	IDDM[a]	[36]
hIns/IFN-γ	IDDM	[36]
rIns/E^d_α,E^b_β	IDDM	[37]
rIns/H-$2K^b$	IDDM	[38]

[a] IDDM = Insulin-dependent diabetes mellitus.

Table 2 lists other animal models of human pathology which have been produced using transgenic mice. Probably the most significant example is the recent production of transgenic mice for human immunodeficiency virus (HIV) (J. Abramczuk *et al.*, pers. comm.). The phenotypic manifestations observed in the transgenic mice were similar to the clinical abnormalities reported in AIDS patients. This includes lymphadenopathy, interstitial pneumonia, psorioform skin lesions and immunological deficiencies. This animal model should be useful for studying the pathogenesis of AIDS and assessing potential therapies.

Gene therapy

Although direct manipulation of embryos would be unlikely to represent the most suitable technique for gene therapy in man, several reports have appeared in the last few years indicating remarkable success in curing genetic diseases in transgenic mice (Table 3).

Several approaches have been employed to replace defective genes. Some will probably hold out more potential than others and they are connected with somatic gene therapy, that is, the removal of human cells, transfection of appropriate genes and their subsequent replacement. Currently the retroviral vectors field is the most active. Dzierzal *et al.* [49] have inserted intact human β-globin genes into several retroviral constructs. It appears that, after injection of stem cells transfected with these vectors into lethally irradiated mice the human globin genes are expressed only in erythroid cells of the recipient for a period ranging from four to nine months.

The major problem of these experiments is the low level of expression. However, Grosveld *et al.* [50] have shown that sequences located 50 Kb upstream and 20 Kb downstream of the human β-globin genes significantly

Table 3. Gene therapy

Construct	Pathological state (correction)	Reference
Mouse or human β globin	Murine β-thalassemia	[44]
mMT-1/r GH	Mouse dwarfism	[45]
E^k_α	E_α-deficiency	[46]
GnRH	Hypogonadism	[47]
MBP	Shiverer	[48]

E^k_α = E complex of MHC (major histocompatibility complex).
GnRH = Gonadotropin releasing hormone.
MBP = Myelin basic protein.

increase their expression in transgenic mice containing a single copy of the sequences. Thus, it should be possible to construct an ideal vector to obtain tissue-specificity and a high level of expression of the human β-globin.

Conclusions and prospectives

We have discussed only a few of the many problems in biology that can be addressed and explored by *in vivo* gene transfer. New tools are not available to increase the rate of isolation of new genes and definition of controlling elements. Transgenic animals will provide valuable experimental models to address fundamental questions of developmental gene expression, immune surveillance, neurobiology, oncogenesis and pathogenesis of diseases.

At present, it is impossible to conceive that alternatives will completely replace animals in biomedical research. *In vitro* and *in vivo* experimentation should be synergistic and be used in parallel by scientists if the aim is that of biomedical progress.

References

1. Gordon JW, Ruddle FH (1983) Gene transfer into mouse embryos: production of transgenic mice by pronuclear injection. *Methods Enzym* 101C: 411–433
2. Palmiter RD, Brinster RL (1985) Transgenic mice. *Cell* 41: 343–345
3. Hogan B, Costantini F, Lacy L (1986) *Manipulating mouse embryo. A Laboratory Manual.* Cold Spring Harbor Lab. Cold Spring Harbor, N.Y.
4. Brinster RL, Palmiter RD (1986) *Introduction of genes into germ line of animals.* Harvey Lect. Alan R. Liss Inc. N.Y. pp 1–38
5. Palmiter RD, Brinster RL, Hammer RE, Trumbaner ME, Rosenfeld MG, Birnberg NC, Evans R (1982) Dramatic growth of mice that develop from eggs microinjected with metallothionein-growth hormone fusion genes. *Nature* 300: 611–615
6. Palmiter RD, Norstedt G, Gelnias RE, Hammer RE, Brinster RL (1983) Metallothionein-Human GH fusion gene stimulate growth of mice. *Science* 222: 809–814
7. Hammer RE, Brinster RL, Rosenfeld MG, Evans RE, Mayo KE (1985) Expression of human growth hormone-releasing factor in transgenic mice results in increased somatic growth. *Nature*

315: 413–416
8. Low MJ, Hammer RE, Goodman RH, Habener JF, Palmiter RD, Brinster RL (1985) Tissue-specific posttranslation processing of pre-prosomatostatin encoded by a metallothionein-somatostatin fusion gene in transgenic mice. *Cell* 41: 211–219
9. Low MJ, Lecham RM, Hammer RE, Brinster RL, Hebener JF, Mandell G, Goodman RH (1986) Gonadotroph-specific expression of metallothionein fusion genes in pituitaries of transgenic mice. *Science* 231: 1002–1004
10. Beamer WG, Eicher EM (1976) Stimulation of growth in the little mouse. *J. Endocrinol.* 71: 37–45
11. Norstedt G, Palmiter RD (1984) Secretory rhythm of growth hormone regulates sexual differentiation of mouse liver. *Cell* 36: 805–812
12. Rivier J, Spiess J, Thorner M, Vale W (1982) Characterization of growth hormone-releasing factor from a human pancreatic islet tumor. *Nature* 300: 276–278
13. Gordon JW (1986) A foreign dehydrofolate reductase gene in transgenic mice acts as a dominant mutation. *Mol Cell Biol* 6: 2158–2167
14. Hoeffler JP, Boockfor FR, Frawley LS (1985) Ontogeny of prolactin cells in neonatal rats: Initial prolactin secretors also release growth hormone. *Endocrinology* 117: 187–195
15. Behringer RR, Mathews LS, Palmiter RD, Brinster RL (1988) Dwarf mice produced by genetic ablation of growth hormone-expressing cells. *Genes and Devel* 2: 453–461
16. Brinster RL, Chen HY, Messing A, van Dyke T, Levine AJ, Palmiter RD (1984) Transgenic mice harboring SV40 T-antigen genes develop characteristic brain tumor. *Cell* 37: 367–379
17. Palmiter RD, Chen HY, Messing A, Brinsker RL (1985) SV40 enhancer and large T-antigen are instrumental in development of choroid plexus tumors in transgenic mice. *Nature* 316: 457–460
18. Small JA, Blair DG, Showalter SD, Scangos GA (1985) Analysis of a transgenic mouse containing simian virus 40 and v-myc sequences. *Mol Cell Biol* 5: 642–648
19. Ornitz DM, Palmiter RD, Messing A, Hammer RE, Pinkert CA, Brinster RL (1985) Elastase I promoter directs expression of human growth hormone and SV40 T-antigen genes to pancreatic acinar cells in transgenic mice. Cold Spring Harbor Symp. *Quant Biol* 50: 399–409
20. Hanahan D (1985) Heritable formation of pancreatic β-cell tumors in transgenic mice expressing recombinant insulin/simian virus 40 oncogenes. *Nature* 315: 115–122
21. Messing A, Chen HY, Palmiter RD, Brinster RL (1985) Peripheral neuropaties, hepatocellular carcinomas, and islet cell adenomas in transgenic mice. *Nature* 316: 461–463
22. Kelly F, Kellermann O, Mechali F, Gaillard J, Babinet C (1986) Expression of simian virus 40 oncogene in F9 embryonal carcinoma cells, in transgenic mice and in transgenic embryos. In Cancer Cells, Vol. IV. Cold Spring Harbor Lab. Cold Spring Harbor, N.Y. pp 263–273
23. Mahon KA, Chepelinsky AB, Khillan JS, Overbeek PA, Piatigorsky J, Westphal H (1987) Oncogenesis of the lens in transgenic mice. *Science* 235: 1622–1628
24. Adams JM, Harris AW, Pinkert CA, *et al.* (1985) The c-myc oncogene driven by immunoglobulin enhancer induces lymphoid malignancy in transgenic mice. *Nature* 318: 533–538
25. Stewart TA, Pattengale PK, Leder P (1984) Spontaneous mammary adenocarcinomas in transgenic mice that carry and express MTV/myc fusion genes. *Cell* 38: 627–637
26. Quaife CJ, Pinkert CA, Ornitz DM, Palmiter RD, Brinster RL (1987) Pancreatic neoplasia induced by ras expression in acinar cells of transgenic mice. *Cell* 48: 1023–1034
27. Sinn E, Muller W, Pattengale P, Tepler I, Wallace R, Leder P (1987) Coexpression of MMTV/V-Ha-ras and MMTV/c-myc genes in transgenic mice: Synergistic action of oncogenes in vivo. *Cell* 49: 466–475
28. Andres A-C, Schönenberger C-A, Grouer B, Henninghausen L, Le Meur M, Gerlinger P (1987) Ha-ras oncogene expression directed by a milk protein gene promoter: tissue specificity, hormonal regulation, and tumor induction in transgenic mice. *Proc Natl Acad Sci* (USA) 84: 1299–1303
29. Bautch VL, Toda S, Hassel JA, Hanahan D (1987) Endothelial cell tumors develop in transgenic mice carrying polyoma virus middle T oncogene. *Cell* 51: 529–538

30. Lacey ML, Albert S, Hanahan D (1986) The bovine papilloma virus genome elicits skin tumors in transgenic mice. *Nature* 322: 609–612
31. Small JA, Khoury G, Jay G, Howley PM, Scangos GA (1986) Early region of JC virus and BK virus induce distinct and tissue-specific tumors in transgenic mice. *Proc Natl Acad Sci* (USA) 83: 8288–8292
32. Nerenberg M, Hinrichs SH, Reynolds RK, Khoury G, Jay G (1987) The *tat* gene of human T-lymphotropic virus type I induces mesenchymal tumors in transgenic mice. *Science* 237: 1324–1329
33. ZuRhein GM, Chou S (1965) Particles resembling papova viruses in human demyelinating disease. *Science* 148: 1477
34. Low PA, McCloud JG (1975) Hereditary demyelinating neuropathy in trembler mouse. *J. Neurol. Sci.* 26: 265
35. Hinrichs SH, Nerenberg M, Reynolds RK, Khoury G, Jay G (1987) A transgenic mice model for human neurofibromatosis. *Science* 237: 1340–1343
36. Sartvetnick N, Liggitt D, Pitts SL, Hansen SE, Stewart TA (1988) Insulin-dependent diabetes mellitus induced in transgenic mice by ectopic expression of Class II MHC and Interferon-gamma. *Cell* 52: 773–782
37. Lo D, Burkey LC, Widera G, *et al.* (1988) Diabetes and tolerance in transgenic mice expressing Class II molecules in pancreatic beta cells. *Cell* 53: 159–168
38. Allison J, Campbell IL, Moraham G, Mandel TE, Harrison LC, Miller JFAP (1988) Diabetes in transgenic mice resulting from over-expression of Class I histocompatibility molecules in pancreatic β cells. *Nature* 333: 529–533
39. Wagner TE, Hoppe PC, Jollick JD, Scholl DR, Hodinka RL, Gault JB (1981) Microinjection of a rabbit β-globin gene into zygotes and its subsequent expression. *Proc Natl Acad Sci* (USA) 78: 6373–6380
40. Sasaki H, Shigenobu T, Nakazatu M, *et al.* (1986) Generation of transgenic mice producing a human transthyretin variant: a possible mouse model for familial amyloidotic polyneuropathy. *Biochem Biophys Res Comm* 139: 794–799
41. Hooper M, Hardy K, Handyside A, Hunter S, Monk M (1987) HPHT-deficient (Lesch-Nyhan) mouse embryos derived from germline colonization by cultured cells. *Nature* 326: 292–295
42. Rüther U, Garber C, Komitowski D, Muller R, Wagner EF (1987) Deregulated c-fos expression interferes with normal bone development in transgenic mice. *Nature* 325: 412–416
43. Katsuki M, Sato M, Kimura M, Yokoyama M, Kobayashi, Nomura T (1988) Conversion of normal behaviour to shiverer by myelin basic protein antisense cDNA in transgenic mice. *Science* 241: 593–595
44. Costantini F, Chada K, Magram J (1986) Correction of murine β-thalassemia by gene transfer into the germ line. *Science* 233: 1192–1194
45. Hammer RE, Palmiter RD, Brinster RL (1984) Partial correction of murine hereditary disorder by germ-line incorporation of a new gene. *Nature* 311: 65–67
46. Le Meur M, Gerlinger P, Benoist C, Mathis D (1985) Correcting an immuno-response deficiency by creating E_α gene transgenic mice. *Nature* 316: 38–42
47. Mason AJ, Pitt SL, Nikolics K, *et al.* (1986) The hypogonadal mouse: reproductive functions restored by gene therapy. *Science* 234: 1372–1378
48. Readhead C, Popko B, Takanashi N, *et al.* (1987) Expression of a myelin basic protein gene in transgenic shiverer mice: correction of the dysmyelinating phenotype. *Cell* 48: 703–712
49. Dzierzak EA, Papayannopoulou T, Mulligan RC (1988) Lineage-specific expression of a human β-globin gene in murine reconstituted with retrovirus-transduced stem cells. *Nature* 331: 35–41
50. Grosveld F, van Assendelff G, Greaves D, Kollias G (1988) *Cell* (in press)

[illegible]

39. Wagner TE, Hoppe PC, Jollick JD, Scholl DR, Hodinka RL, Gault JB (1981) Microinjection of a rabbit β-globin gene into zygotes and its subsequent expression [illegible]

[illegible]

42. Rüther U, Garber C, Komitowski D, Müller R, Wagner EF (1987) Deregulated c-fos expression interferes with normal bone development in transgenic mice. Nature 325: 412-416

43. [illegible] (1988) [illegible]

44. Costantini F, Chada K, Magram J (1986) Correction of murine β-thalassemia by gene transfer into the germ line. Science 233: 1192-1194

45. Hammer RE, Palmiter RD, Brinster RL (1984) Partial correction of murine hereditary growth disorder by germ-line incorporation of a new gene. Nature 311: 65-67

46. Le Meur M, Gerlinger P, Benoist C, Mathis D (1985) Correcting an immune-response deficiency by creating Eα gene transgenic mice. Nature 316: 38-42

47. Mason AJ, Pitts SL, Nikolics K, et al. (1986) The hypogonadal mouse: reproductive functions restored by gene therapy. Science 234: 1372-1378

48. Readhead C, Popko B, Takahashi N, et al. (1987) Expression of a myelin basic protein gene in transgenic shiverer mice: correction of the dysmyelinating phenotype. Cell 48: 703-712

49. [illegible]

50. [illegible] (1988) [illegible] (in press)

Recent progress toward reducing the use of animal experimentation in biomedical research

MICHAEL BALLS
Fund for the Replacement of Animals in Medical Experiments (FRAME), Department of Human Morphology, University of Nottingham Medical School, Nottingham, UK

Introduction

Before I begin to address the subject of this article, some background points need to be made, so that the reader can evaluate my role in this Symposium.

Although I am employed as a full-time teacher, researcher and administrator in the University of Nottingham Medical School, I also devote much of my time to acting in effect, as honorary director of *FRAME* (Fund for the Replacement of Animals in Medical Experiments). FRAME is a Three Rs organisation in the *reduction*, *refinement*, *replacement* tradition established by Russell & Burch [1] and we have adopted a Three Rs definition of *alternatives*, based on that proposed by Professor David Smyth in his excellent book on this subject [2], to include:

> all procedures which can completely replace the need for animal experiments, reduce the numbers of animals required, or diminish the amount of pain and distress suffered by animals in meeting the essential needs of man and other animals.

The term *alternative* has come to have a special meaning in this context, and is now widely accepted internationally, for example, in the 1986 US Office of Technology Assessment report on *Alternatives to Animal Use in Research, Education and Testing* [3], and the 1988 US National Research Council report on the *Use of Laboratory Animals in Biomedical and Behavioural Research* [4]. I think the time is over for promoting the terms *ancillary*, *adjunct*, *additive* or *complementary* to describe replacement alternative methods as almost all concerned recognise the usefulness of this definition, despite its apparent etymological limitations.

FRAME is both a human welfare *and* an animal welfare organisation, and we reject any suggestion that there is no alternative other than to be *either* for humans *or* for animals. Our approach is not an easy one to sustain, for we are constantly under pressure from antivivisectionists on the one hand, and from the more libertarian animal experimenters on the other, to move closer to *their* positions. I survive by adhering to my own golden rule – I never tailor my views, or my talks, to suit particular audiences, so I often

S. Garattini (ed.), The Importance of Animal Experimentation for Safety and Biomedical Research, 223–235.

feel isolated. That can require courage – it is no alibi.

FRAME could not exist without the support and encouragement given by scientists and others in universities, research institutions, industrial companies and governments in many countries. They are editors of our journal, *ATLA* (Alternatives to Laboratory Animals), they are members of the FRAME Toxicity Committee and the FRAME Research Advisory Committee, they help fund many of our activities, and we work with them in research on the development of valid replacement alternative methods.

My own motivation is that of a common-sense moralist of the protestant Christian tradition, and I fall into the benevolent utilitarian category (number 4) outlined by Timothy Sprigge [5]. But I have to say that I reject most of the ideas and conclusions expressed by Carl Cohen [6]. The central question is not one of human and animal 'rights', but of human *responsibilities*. Over-emotional arguments are frequently used in favour of animal experiments, as well as against them.

I will not deal with refinement and replacement in this presentation, as I will concentrate on the search for a reduction in animal experiments by questioning and evaluating their necessity and their acceptability.

Reasons for reducing animal experiments

I believe that there are powerful ethical and scientific reasons for reducing, limiting, and eventually replacing altogether, the use of animals as surrogates for human beings in laboratory experiments:

Morality

It is the duty of human being to behave more properly toward one another, other animals, other living organisms and, indeed, the world as a whole. Concerns for human welfare, animal welfare and the protection of the environment go hand in hand.

Compassion

Suffering as a result of pain, distress, deprivation and confinement is caused, unavoidably and avoidably, in experiments on animals.

Conservation

The use of wild-caught members of endangered species as laboratory animals can contribute to their likely absence from the world of the future.

Scientific

Animal experiments can be misleading, because of species differences, and the relevance of the information they provide, as in some routine toxicity tests, cannot be accurately known.

Economics

Animal experiments can be very wasteful of human and financial resources.

Politics

There is growing public concern, sometimes justifiable outrage, at what is done to animals in the name of biomedical science. I can see no prospect that this legitimate concern will lessen in the future. Many responsible organisations, such as FRAME, will do all they can to ensure that it does not.

Laws

New national and international legislation, such as the British *Animals (Scientific Procedures) Act 1986* [7] and the 1986 EC Directive on the *Approximation of Laws, Regulations and Administrative Provisions of the Member States Regarding the Protection of Animals Used for Experimental and Other Scientific Purposes* [8], require that animal experimentation is reduced, refined and replaced wherever possible, and that its necessity is justified. I applaud the introduction of these excellent laws and, sadly, there are many recent examples which show that equally strong legislation is necessary in other countries and other parts of the world.

These laws set a framework of sensible controls, and should rarely lead to litigation - only lawyers, certainly not animals or science, would stand to gain from that. However, the possibility of conflict with the requirements of other laws (e.g. on toxicity testing) must be recognised [9].

The question, then, is not *whether* experiments on living vertebrate animals should be controlled, but *how* they should be controlled. In particular, what should be allowed and what should not, and what specific limitations should be applied to the use of particular procedures or particular species.

The defence of animal experiments

Animal experiments are carried out, and defended, for five main reasons:

Education and training

An essential understanding of the structure and functions of the parts of the vertebrate body cannot be gained in any other way.

Fundamental research

Effective means for preventing and treating human (and animal) disease require greater knowledge of organs and systems, as well as at the molecular and cellular levels.

Discovery of biologically active compounds

The discovery and efficacy evaluation of drugs intended for human use has required, and will continue to require, the use of animal models.

Production of useful biological materials

Whole animals are essential for the production of useful molecules, such as antibodies, including monoclonal antibodies.

Toxicity testing and safety testing

Evaluation of the potential hazard of exposure to chemical compounds, chemical formulations and other materials requires tests in the whole body, especially as a means of detecting unexpected effects.

The principal underlying reason is, of course, that human beings are prepared to use animals in ways which would not be ethically acceptable if applied to each other. Nevertheless, I recognise that useful knowledge of one kind or another has been gained from animal experimentation.

Necessity

In considering why 4.5 million experiments on animals were begun in the UK in 1984, Sir William Paton, a distinguished pharmacologist, wrote, 'The answer can only be that that is the number that was found necessary' [10]. I consider this to be a weak line of argument, for animal experiments cannot be justified in terms of logical or mathematical necessity, conceptual or analytic necessity, or causal necessity, but only by *conditional* necessity [11].

What follows is that, whether or not the claim of necessity is acceptable, it depends on other matters and involves value judgements. Assessment of such a claim involves two stages [11]. First, is the proposed course of action the only means to the desired end? That is, is there no alternative way involving fewer animals, less sentient animals, less painful procedures, or non-animal methods? Consideration of these questions is required by both the 1986 UK Act (ASPA) and the 1986 EC Directive (ECD):

ASPA (5.5): The Secretary of State shall not grant a project licence unless he is satisfied that the applicant has given adequate consideration to the feasibility of achieving the purpose of the programme to be specified in the licence by means not involving the use of protected animals.

ECD (7.2): An experiment shall not be performed if another scientifically satisfactory method of obtaining the result sought, not entailing the use of an animal, is reasonably and practicably available.

ECD (7.3): When an experiment has to be performed, the choice of species shall be carefully considered and, where necessary, explained to the authority. In a choice between experiments, those which use the minimum number of animals, involve animals with the lowest degree of neurophysiological sensitivity, cause the least pain, suffering, distress or lasting harm and which are most likely to provide satisfactory results shall be selected.

Another way of phrasing this quotation is to ask whether a particular procedure is necessary in the sense of *essential* (i.e. there can be no other way) or merely *sufficient* (i.e. other ways are also possible). The position can change with time. For example, primary cultures of monkey kidney cells were once the only way of producing polio vaccine. Now it can be done with cultured human cells. So what was once essential has become only sufficient – and the case for killing monkeys to obtain their kidneys is thereby weakened.

The second stage requires evaluation of the grounds on which pursuance of the 'necessary' means is considered justified, and common grounds [12] are that it is:

- *indispensable*, for something else to be achieved (e.g. for the accumulation of fundamental scientific knowledge);
- *imperative*, because of something of higher priority (e.g. overcoming the suffering caused by cancer, heart disease, multiple sclerosis, etc.);
- *requisite*, because of laws or policy decisions, e.g. that new chemicals must be tested in animals before human beings are exposed to them.

Thus, particular animal experiments are only *necessary* if there is no other way of gaining the information they can provide, and if the reasons for requiring that information are convincing. The British Government emphasised the importance of necessity in preparing the way for the 1986 Act [13]:

Animal experiments that are unnecessary, use unnecessarily large numbers of animals, or are unnecessarily painful are indefensible.

The operation of these principles requires judgement and discrimination in considering an immense range of different circumstances. Generalisation, and especially generalisation from the particular, are the enemies of rational thought and action, here as in many other situations.

The weighing of benefit and suffering

Central to the British Act is the following requirement:

ASPA (5.4): In determining whether and on what terms to grant a project licence the Secretary of State shall weigh the likely adverse effects on the animals concerned against the benefit likely to accrue as a result of the programme to be specified in the licence.

I wholeheartedly support this principle. However, it represents an area of weakness and uncertainty at present, and unless we deal with this problem, the Act will not be as effective as was anticipated.

Benefit

That the animal experimentation of the past has led to great benefits for human beings and other animals has been the dominant theme of this Symposium. Professor Sprigge accepted it, with reservations [5]. Professor Cohen went further, for he said that the good which has resulted outweighs the evil by an *incalculable* (i.e. very large) amount [6]. He also said that virtually every important step in medicine was only possible because of experiments on animals.

This view is central to the NRC report [4] and was earlier discussed at great length by Sir William Paton [10], who asked readers of his book to apply the 'test of deletion' – i.e. to identify what we know as the result of a particular animal experiment, then to calculate what the loss would have been if that experiment had not been done. A classic example is the discovery of insulin as a result of Banting and Best's experiments on a small number of dogs.

Sir William makes many other significant remarks. For example, he expresses a view echoed by Professor Cohen and others at this Symposium, 'As in other matters, our confidence in future benefit is a function of the historical record'. However, Sir William also says that it is dangerous to be too preoccupied with benefit, for knowledge for its own sake 'has a kind of inevitable priority, and our confidence in the expected benefit depends on the soundness of the knowledge'. He goes on to write of 'limited experiments and unlimited benefits'.

These views of historical events are not accepted by everyone. For example, various authors, e.g. Hans Ruesch in *Naked Empress* [14] and Dr Robert Sharpe in *The Cruel Deception* [15], have sought to minimise the significance of animal experiments in the improvement of the quality and length of human life which has undoubtedly taken place during the last 100 years or so.

I reject both these biased attempts to manipulate the contribution made by animal experiments in the past to support a particular viewpoint. I also consider that Sir William's deletion test is unsound. All historians are tempted to ask what would have happened if a particular event had not taken place. The answer is that they cannot know, and they can only guess whether the consequences would have been better or worse than those which actually followed. Thus, I do not accept that insulin would not have been discovered without the work of Banting and Best.

The second weakness of the historical approach is that it sees the future merely as an extension of the past. However, biomedical research and clinical practice are being revolutionised by recent developments, such as monoclonal antibodies, NMR imaging, gene detection by RFLPs, gene cloning and gene transfer, computer graphics and drug design, to name but a few. Should we assume that there will not be equally surprising new developments in the future? Also, there are already many substantial discoveries which *could only* have been found through the use of non-animal methods. Therefore, I believe that the current reliance on animal experimentation will be steadily reduced, and that it will one day be possible to take drugs from the design stages via non-animal alternatives to the patient - without any use of animals. The only question is, how soon?

In the immediate future, however, there is a need for the formulation of objective ways of quantitatively assessing the likely benefit to be gained from a particular course of proposed animal-based research. Otherwise, what can we put on the benefit side of the benefit-suffering equation? At the very least, then, we must find ways of assessing both the degree of benefit which might accrue, and the probability that that such benefit would accrue. We could begin by trying to think in terms of three main categories: *low*, *medium* and *high* probability of significant benefit.

Suffering

Since what became known as the *Cruelty to Animals Act* was passed in Britain in 1876 [16], there has been much discussion about *pain* and its assessment. That is part of the reason why *suffering*, which also includes distress, discomfort, deprivation and confinement, was the term used in the 1986 Act. For example, while we do not know whether chimpanzees experience pain as a result of being housed in isolation in small metal cages, they undoubtedly suffer as a result of deprivation, confinement and lack of close contact with other members of their own species.

In both Britain and the Netherlands, suffering is considered and categorised as of *mild*, *moderate* or *substantial* severity. The criteria for the assessment of suffering have not yet been fully worked out or agreed, but the problem is currently being given much attention (e.g. [17]). There seems to be greater reluctance in Britain than in the Netherlands to place procedures in the substantial category. Another problem is overuse of the moderate category, and in Britain we are already talking of the low end and the high end of moderate - so, given that there must also be a middle part of this band, we may already have five categories!

Weighing the balance

Agreeing on ways of assessing potential/likely benefit and suffering is a matter of the highest priority, but we must also consider how to weigh the balance between these assessments of two different phenomena - and who should do it.

At a superficial level, it would be obvious that if likely benefit was assessed as high and suffering low, then the work should be allowed. Similarly, if the likely benefit was assessed as low and suffering high, then no project licence should be given. However, where both benefit and suffering were considered likely to be substantial, then very careful consideration and judgement would be needed, including a rigorous assessment of the quality of the science. Indeed, Professor Patrick Bateson [18] has suggested that *quality*

Table 1. Criteria for judging a basic research project

1. The applicants and their laboratory:
   - general standing of the laboratory
   - reputations of scientists
   - quality of animal care facilities
   - quality of animal technicians and named persons
2. The proposed project work:
   - originality of concepts
   - relevance of goals of the research
   - understanding of background
   - quality of working hypothesis
   - quality of plan of work
   - necessity in view of other work in progress in the field
3. The procedures to be used:
   - relevance of procedures
   - standard of equipment available
   - evidence of experience with procedures
   - quality of plans for anaesthesia, analgesia, and general after-care
4. Animal welfare aspects:
   - genuine awareness of animal welfare issues
   - care in choice of species
   - sincerity of attempts at:
     - reduction in numbers to be used
     - refinement of procedures to minimise suffering
     - replacement by non-animal methods
5. Overall assessment:
   - ratings in three categories (low, medium, high):
     a. quality of applicant and laboratory
     b. quality of proposed project work
     c. necessity of procedures to be used
     d. potential/likely scientific benefit
     e. sincerity of animal welfare consideration
     f. potential/likely animal suffering

of science should be brought in as a third consideration. Thus, for example, potential benefit could be high, but only if the quality of the scientific hypothesis were also high. Grantgiving bodies already have systems for evaluating scientific merit. Jacqueline Southee and I have recently put forward some suggested criteria for use in evaluating fundamental research projects [19], summarised in Table 1.

The British Act relies heavily on a full-time inspectorate and a part-time advisory committee to give advice to the responsible Government minister. Both groups can appoint expert assessors. The Animal Procedures Committee in Britain includes members principally interested in animal welfare, as well as lawyers, scientists, doctors and veterinarians. Regional or institutional ethical and/or scientific review committees are used in other countries.

Although I see this approach (along with the greatest possible effort to develop valid non-animal replacement alternatives) as the way forward, it has two unavoidable consequences. First, those committed to the animal welfare movement must recognise that some animal experiments will be permitted, including some whose procedures involve substantial severity. Secondly, those principally interested in scientific and medical progress must recognise that certain current-acceptable procedures will no longer be permitted, even though the potential benefit from them would be substantial.

If these consequences are recognised and accepted, then, as Professor Bateson has pointed out [18], a very big step forward would be taken in achieving an effective 'set of controls to take into account both the interests of what is best in science and those of the animals used in research'.

Strategies for reducing animal experiments

The strategies to be used in seeking a reduction in the scale of animal experimentation must depend on the purposes for which the experiments are proposed.

Reducing animal experimentation in education and training

The EC Directive and the new British Act prohibit animal experimentation by individuals below a certain age, but so-called scientific research projects still lead to appalling and unacceptable suffering in schools in other parts of the world, such as the USA [19]. This problem has been the focus of a campaign by Dr Barbara Orlans at the Scientists Center for Animal Welfare [20], but was very weakly addressed in the OTA Report [3].

Many consider that the use of animal experimentation in practical classes in first-degree science and medicine courses cannot be justified, especially as many graduates now take up careers outside science [21]. This even applies to graduates in pharmacy, pharmacology and the agricultural and veterinary sciences. Medical students at Nottingham University are not required to carry out animal experiments at any stage of their training.

Special courses, involving consideration of the ethical issues involved, as well as the proper care and handling of animals, should be mandatory for those who must use animal experimentation in their special undergraduate project or postgraduate research.

Reducing animal experimentation in fundamental research

As has already been discussed, basic research presents one of the biggest challenges to moderate reformers, since it is at present too easy for biomedical research scientists to use the historical record and vague promises of benefit to justify their projects. Often, they are also able to give scant recognition to the concept of replacement alternatives, before stating that none are available for their own work. This is an area where the benefit/science/suffering analysis should be most rigorously applied, but this will only be possible after agreement has been reached on how it should be done.

Discovery of biologically active compounds

Animal use has already been significantly reduced in research for new drug discovery, where drug design on the basis of molecular and cell biology, biochemistry and computer graphics has replaced the empirical, 'Let's put this compound in the animal to see what happens' approach. These trends will continue, with smaller numbers of animals being used, for the time being, for later-stage efficacy testing.

Production of biologically active molecules

Although antisera have been produced from animals for a long while, two relatively new developments give cause for concern. First, although monoclonal antibodies can be produced *in vitro*, it is said to be easier to produce them from animals. Considerable suffering is involved, and more determined efforts to improve the *in vitro* systems should be encouraged. Secondly, the genetic engineering of animals and the patenting of the animals produced raise to new ethical questions. As in the case of experiments on aborted human embryos, there is a danger that society will be presented with a scientific *fait accompli* that is, the procedures will be developed and in operation, and the 'benefits' will be there for us all to see, before moral consequences have been addressed by those who have a right to know what is going on and to influence policy.

Toxicity testing

Although toxicity tests are ostensibly carried out for the protection of human beings, animals and the environment, animals continue to be used in unnecessarily large numbers, in unnecessarily painful procedures and for the unnecessary testing of unnecessary products. The nightmare jungle of regulatory guidelines is an international scandal and, even when some degree of harmonisation is achieved, agreed guidelines can be operated in nationalistic ways.

As Gerhard Zbinden has recently pointed out [22], many of the guidelines have not been subjected to adequate scientific scrutiny, sometimes it is impossible to follow them, and regulators have almost totally failed to pay any attention to animal welfare issues.

The FRAME Toxicity Committee reported on this issue in 1983 [23], and their recommendations were given prominent consideration in the OTA Report [3]. A second FRAME report will be published in 1990. Meanwhile, one cannot escape the conclusion that, while toxicity testing must be made more scientific and more humane, the blocks on progress are mainly *political*. The way ahead, then, is for citizens to use their democratic rights and press their elected representatives to see that drastic reforms are achieved. Of particular concern is evidence of demands for *more* toxicity testing. For example, there are proposals within the EC which, if accepted, would require the production of toxicity profiles for thousands of cosmetic ingredients, including the testing to toxic levels of chemicals employed in tiny quantities, which have been in use for decades.

Nevertheless, it is clear from what Dr Tom Connors says in his paper in these proceedings [24], that persistence *can* lead to changes in regulatory guidelines, to the benefit of animals *and* humans.

Conclusions

There are grounds for optimism and pessimism when we consider the current rate of progress toward reducing laboratory animal experimentation.

On the *positive* side, new and stronger laws are being introduced and implemented in many countries, and scientists are becoming more aware of their responsibilities toward the animals in their laboratories. Greater influence and power are being given to those who provide day-to-day care for laboratory animals, and to independent veterinarians who can now by right advise and comment on their well-being and treatment. The Three Rs concept is now widely accepted and there are some genuine efforts toward finding replacement alternative methods. Of particular promise is the requirement that the likely suffering of the animals to be used in a programme of work must be considered, along with the potential benefits likely to accrue to human beings, other animals, and to science in general. We should all welcome and encourage these developments.

On the *negative* side, there is evidence of growing conservatism and resistance to change in parts of the scientific community [4], and the numbers of laboratory animals used in some countries are increasing (e.g. in the USA [25], Japan [26] and the Netherlands [27]. Meanwhile, the genetic engineering of animals raises new ethical problems, and the production of biological materials from genetically-engineered organisms raises new problems of safety and toxicity testing in general, while the harmonisation of national and international testing guidelines remains a dream. Funding is insufficient for the development and validation of alternatives, so it is too easy for scientists to say that the use of animals in their particular research is unavoidable. Moreover, scientists have little trouble in justifying the necessity of their fundamental research, and it is not easy to see how greater stringency can be applied in the short term to assessment of the benefit side of the cost-benefit equation. Finally, procedures applied to animals are too readily judged to be mild or moderate, and the present operation of the severity of suffering banding system must be considered unsatisfactory.

Many of those who belong to what has become known as the moderate animal welfare movement, and who are giving their support to the new legislative controls, are disappointed at the rate of progress being achieved. If the promise of genuine refinement, replacement and, above all *reduction* of animal experimentation is not seen to be realised within the immediate future, it will be their duty to press for further and stronger legislation.

References

1. Russell WMS, Burch RL (1959) *The Principles of Human Experimental Technique*. Methuen, London
2. Smyth DH (1978) *Alternatives to Animal Experiments*. Scolar Press, London
3. Office of Technology Assessment (1988) *Alternatives to Animal Use in Research, Testing and Education*. Marcel Dekker, New York
4. National Research Council (1988) *Use of Laboratory Animals in Biomedical and Behavioural Research*. National Academy Press, Washington DC
5. Sprigge TLS (1989) *The ethics of animal use in biomedicine*. This symposium
6. Cohen C (1989) *Animal Experimentation defended: utilities and rights*. This symposium
7. Animals (Scientific Procedures) Act 1986 (1986) HMSO, London
8. Council Directive of 24 November 1986 on the Approximation of Laws, Regulations and Administrative Provisions of the Member States Regarding the Protection of Animals Used for Experimental and Other Purposes (1986) *Official Journal of the European Communities* 29 (L358): 1–29
9. Environmental Resources Limited (1988) *EEC Directives and Animal Testing*. EUR 11353 EN. European Commission, Brussels-Luxembourg
10. Paton W (1984) *Man and Mouse: Animals in Medical Research*. Oxford University Press, Oxford
11. Balls EM (1988) *Animal experimentation – a necessary evil. FRAME NEWS* 20: 5
12. Rowson RH (1988) *A note on the 'necessity' of using animals in research. ATLA* 15: 311–312
13. Scientific Procedures on Living Animals (1985) Cmnd 9521. HMSO, London
14. Ruesch H (1982) *Naked Empress – or the Great Medical Fraud*. CIVITAS, New York
15. Sharpe R (1988) *The Cruel Deception*. Thorsons, Wellingborough
16. An Act to Amend the Law Relating to Cruelty to Animals (1876) Government Office, London
17. Anon (1987) *Animal Experimentation in The Netherlands. ATLA* 15: 113–114
18. Bateson P (1986) When to experiment on animals. *New Scientist* (20 February 1986), 30–32

19. Balls M, Southee JS (1989) Reducing animal experiments by questioning their necessity. In: D. Paterson (Ed) *The Status of Animals. BVA Animal Welfare Foundation*, London, (in press)
20. Orlans FB (1985) Science fairs – a sampling of misguided experiments. *Animal Welfare Institute Quarterly* 34: 108–111
21. Taylor J (1988) Degrees of salary and satisfaction. *Nature*, London 334: 393–394
22. Zbinden G (1988) A look behind drug regulatory guidelines. In: S Adler, G Zbinden (Eds) *National and International Drug Safety Guidelines*, pp 7–14, M.T.C. Varlag, Zollikon
23. Balls M, Riddell RJ, Worden AN (Eds) (1983) Animals and Alternatives in Toxicity Testing. *Academic Press*, London and New York
24. Connors T (1989) The use of animal models in cancer chemotherapy. This symposium
25. Anon (1988) Laboratory animal use increases. *Animal Welfare Institute Quarterly* 37: 16
26. Anon (1988) Animal use in Japan. *ATLA* 15: 278

Animal use in drug research*

MARTIN KRAMER
Hoechst AG, Frankfurt/Main, FRG

Some 100 years ago experimental drug research in animals started on an industrial scale and the first drugs were antipyrine and acetylsalicylic acid. Experimental chemotherapy of infectious diseases was started by Paul Ehrlich who was able to standardize an animal model, the tryposoma infection of the mouse, which enabled him to detect finally the first compound active against syphilis which was tolerated by the host (Fig. 1) [1]. Compound number 606 finally was the famous Salvarsan known also as Ehrlich Hata 606.

The topic of my paper requires me to come back to history, because until recently some medical doctors and even clinicians with a certain standing

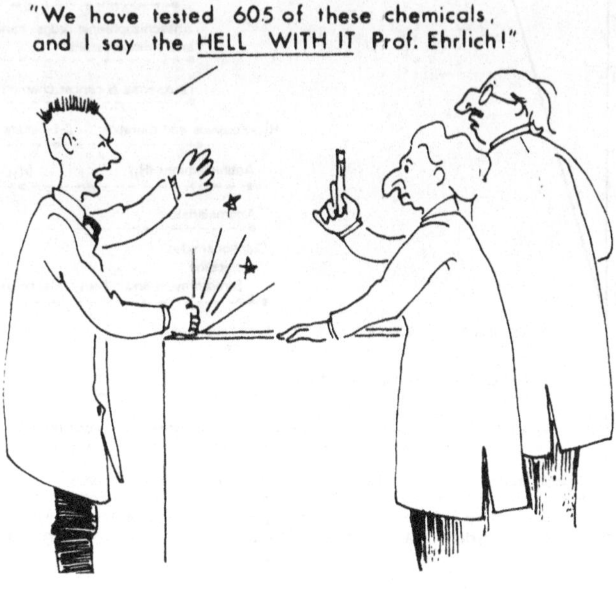
"We have tested 605 of these chemicals, and I say the HELL WITH IT Prof. Ehrlich!"

Fig. 1.

* Dedicated to Prof. Dr. rer. nat. Hansgeorg Gareis on the occasion of his 60th birthday.

S. Garattini (ed.), The Importance of Animal Experimentation for Safety and Biomedical Research, 237–246.

denied the importance of animal experiments in the search of new drugs. This is illustrated by a paper of Burkhardt *et al.* [2] from which I quote some sentences:

It is difficult to predict events with reasonable certainty even within one particular animal species. The problem of extrapolation is being viewed under three different aspects: when there is no previous experience at all,

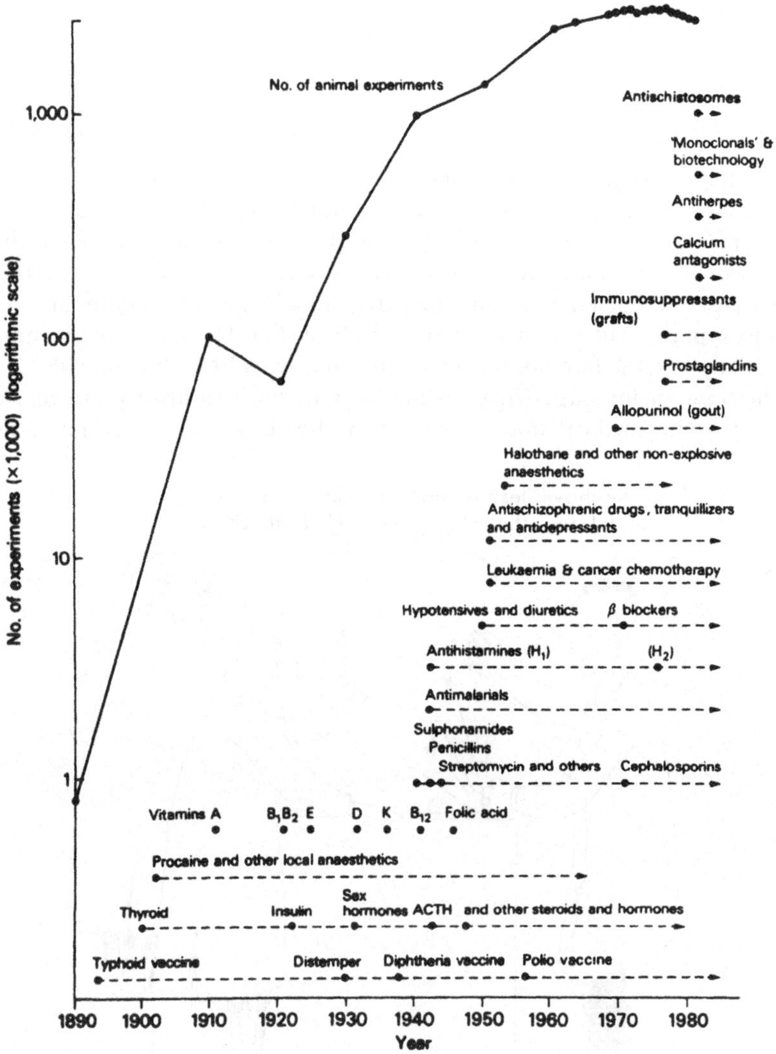

Fig. 2. Animal experiment and medical advance (taken from W. Paton: Man and Mouse). The first letter of the word or phrase describing the advance is set opposite the approximate date of its introduction. Broken lines indicate continued development.

when there is relevant previous experience, and when there are animal models available. In the first case it is impossible to make any prediction at all. In the second case only subjective suppositions are possible. As to the third case it is an open question at the moment whether animal models do exist at all. According to the present state of science it is impossible to make objective predictions for man on the basis of animal trials. Toxicological testing methods allowing the preselection of drugs or any other kind of deduction without verification in man do not exist.

Figure 2 shows the increase of animal experiments in the UK compared to milestones of progress in prophylaxis and therapy particularly coming from drug research (taken from Paton [3]). The number of animal experiments has increased over the years but this increase is connected with considerable progress in the possibilities to treat diseases which formerly could not be cured. Most of these new remedies came directly out of results of animal experiments.

I should like to illustrate this with some examples, the first being calcium antagonists. The first calcium channel blocker was verapamil, a compound which was developed for the treatment of angina and which was found exclusively in animal experiments. Its mode of action, namely to block the voltage-dependent calcium channel, was clarified very much later and only since this mode of action was known has it been possible to develop other compounds of a similar type. The screening for calcium-channel blocking property can now be done of course using *in vitro* methods.

Calcium channel blockers are at the present time widely and increasingly

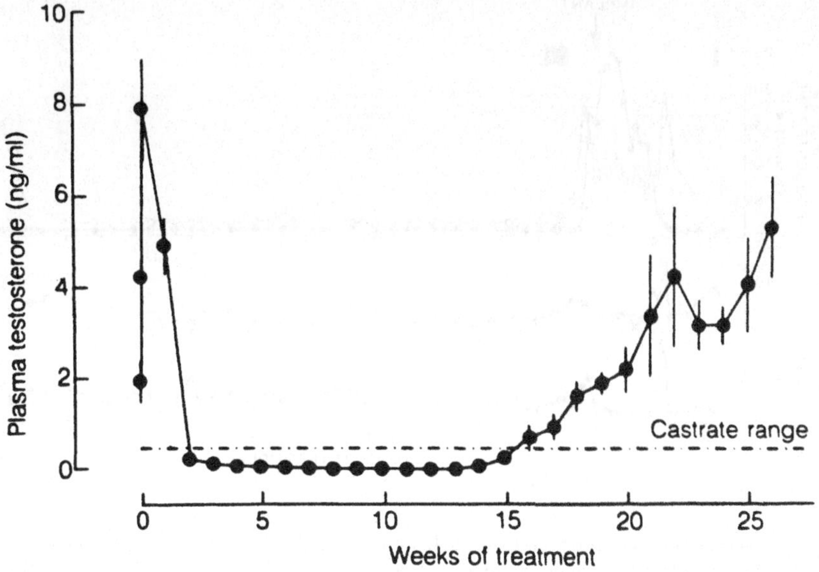

Fig. 3. Plasma testosterone in dogs after treatment with an implant containing 3 mg buserelin.

used for the treatment of hypertension and congestive heart failure.

Another example are the inhibitors of the enzyme that converts angiotensin 1 to angiotensin 2. The first compound active on this converting enzyme was a peptide, a derivative of pepstatin. The usefulness of this principle to inhibit the conversion of angiotensin 1 to angiotensin 2 had first to be established in a number of animal experiments and models before attempts could be made to modify the chemical structure in order to get an orally absorbable ACE-inhibitor. The first result was captopril.

The third example is buserelin, a LH-RH analogue which is about 100 times more active than the natural peptide and which has a longer duration of action. Only in animal experimentations could it be shown that small doses produced a release of gonadotropin whereas larger doses produced a receptor down-regulation within the anterior pituitary with the consequence of an inhibition of LH secretion. The inhibition of gonadotropin secretion was followed by inhibition of steroid biosynthesis in the testes or the ovaries of laboratory animals and man. The compound and its analogues are now successfully used in the treatment of prostate cancer, breast cancer, and endometriosis. Such treatment, particularly with sustained release forms, reduces the testosterone concentration to castration levels and this reduction is reversible when the treatment is discontinued (Fig. 3).

Figure 3 shows testosterone levels in a dog with a subcutaneous buserelin implant (polyactide/glycolide containing 3 mg buserelin). There was an initial rise of testosterone then plasma testosterone remained suppressed for 15 weeks.

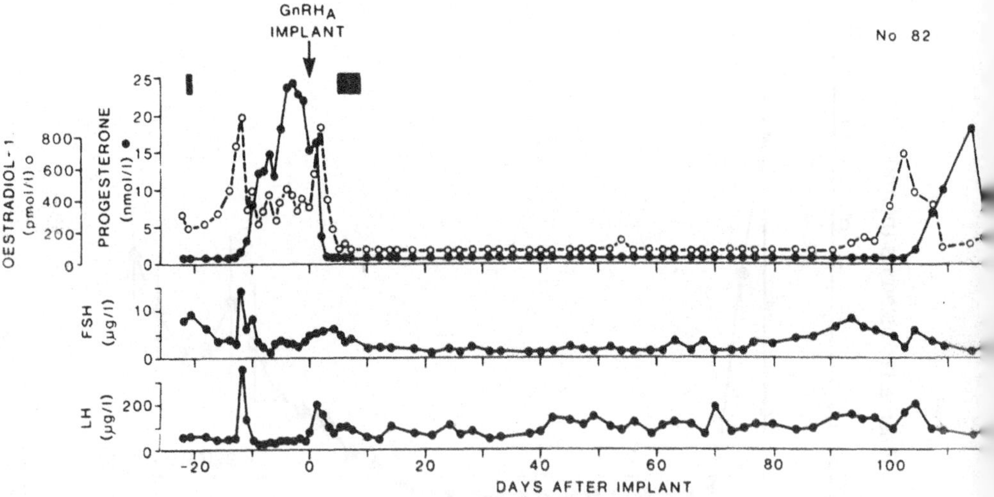

■ Menstrual bleeding.

Fig. 4. Serum concentrations of LH, FSH, estradiol and progesterone in a macaque treated with a PLG implant containing buserelin (arrow). Note that during the recovery phase, the rise in FSH is followed by prompt restoration of ovarian activity.

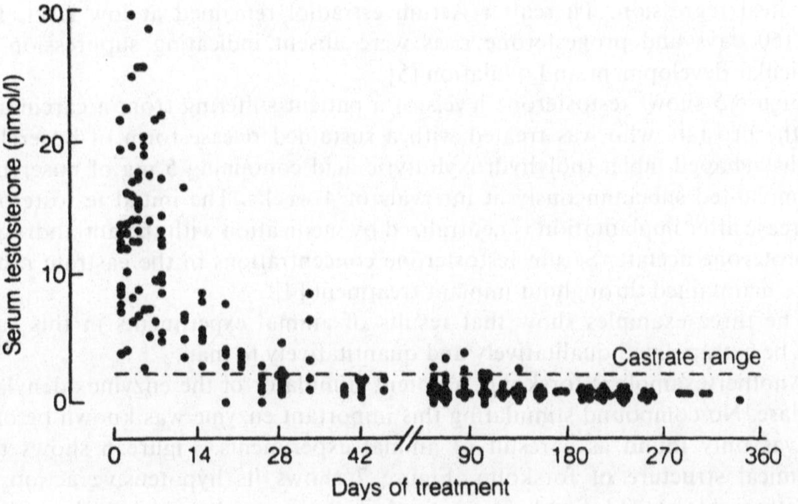

Fig. 5. Serum testosterone in patients with carcinoma of the prostate. A disk shaped tablet containing 5 mg buserelin is implanted subcutaneously at intervals of 4 weeks.

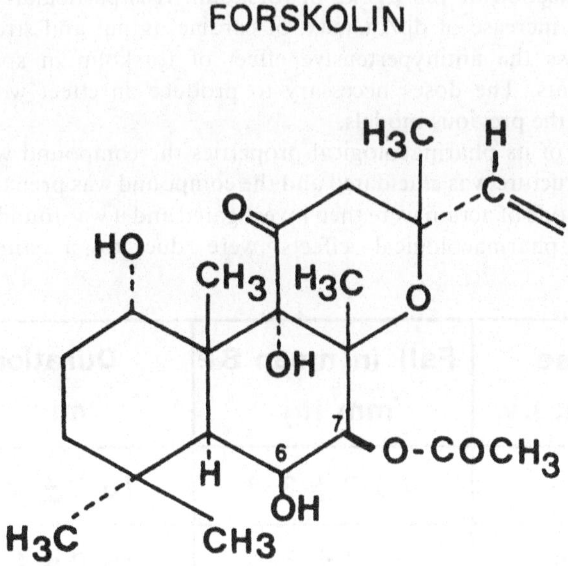

Fig. 6. Chemical structure of forskolin.

After complete release of buserelin testosterone levels returned slowly to normal [4].

Figure 4 shows LH, FSH, estradiol, and progesterone in a macaque treated with a buserelin implant during the luteal phase. Serum progesterone and estradiol concentrations rose for 1–2 days before falling at the expected time of luteal regression. Thereafter, serum estradiol remained at low levels for 90–160 days and progesterone rises were absent indicating suppression of follicular development and ovulation [5].

Figure 5 shows testosterone levels of a patient suffering from a carcinoma of the prostate who was treated with a sustained release form of buserelin. A disk-shaped tablet (polyhydroxybutyric acid containing 5 mg of buserelin) is implanted subcutaneously at intervals of 4 weeks. The initial testosterone increase after implantation is neutralized by medication with the antiandrogen cyproterone acetate. Serum testosterone concentrations in the castrate range were maintained throughout implant treatment [4].

The three examples show that results of animal experiments in this case can be extrapolated qualitatively and quantitatively to man.

Another example is forskolin, a potent stimulator of the enzyme adenylate cyclase. No compound stimulating this important enzyme was known before. It was only found as a result of animal experiments. Figure 6 shows the chemical structure of forskolin. Figure 7 shows its hypotensive action in anesthesized cats [6]. Small amounts of forskolin produce a dose-dependent fall in arterial blood pressure, and its duration was dose-dependent too. Figure 8 shows several pharmacological parameters in the anesthesized dog after intravenous injection of 100 μg/kg of forskolin. It is particularly interesting to see a sharp increase of dp/dt max, of cardiac output and stroke volume. Figure 9 shows the antihypertensive effect of forskolin in spontaneously hypertensive rats. The doses necessary to produce an effect were 20 times higher than in the previous models.

On account of its pharmacological properties the compound was purified, its chemical structure was elucidated and the compound was prepared in larger amounts. Its mode of action were then investigated and it was found by Metzger [7] that all pharmacological effects were due to a stimulation of

Dose μg/kg, i.v.	Fall in mean B.P. mm Hg	Duration min.
50	49·7 ± 3·2	16·7 ± 2·1
100	63·7 ± 5·5	55·0 ± 3·9
250	72·2 ± 6·2	97·5 ± 5·6

Values are mean ± s.e.m.

Fig. 7. Hypotensive action of forskolin in anesthetized cats.

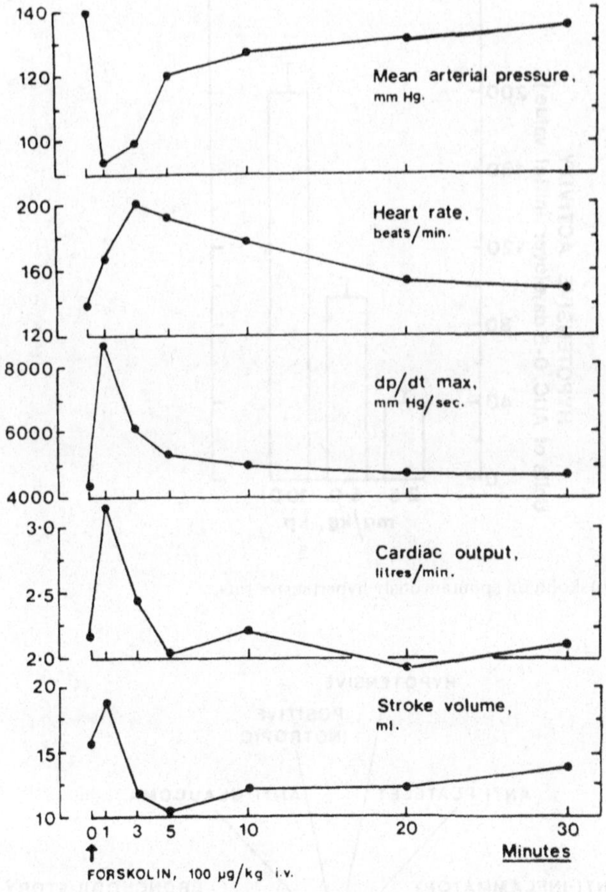

Fig. 8. Effect of forskolin on parameters of circulation on anesthetized dogs.

adenylate cyclase and an increase in cAMP-concentration (Fig. 10).

Figure 11 shows a strong correlation between the increase in contractile force in guinea pig atria and an increase in adenylate cyclase activity and in cAMP-dependent protein kinase. It was furthermore found that forskolin binds to a catalytic subunit of adenylate cyclase and this binding property could be used for the purification of adenylate cyclase by affinity chromatography with forskolin (Fig. 12). By this means adenylate cyclase can be recovered with an enrichment factor up to 2000.

Forskolin is a universal adenylate cyclase activator. It activates cyclases from nearly all tissues tested so far. The only exception seems to be the sperm adenylate cyclase. The binding of forskolin to the cyclase is fast and reversible and it can be removed simply by washing the treated cells of membranes.

Forskolin is a good illustration of the fact that even activities which can

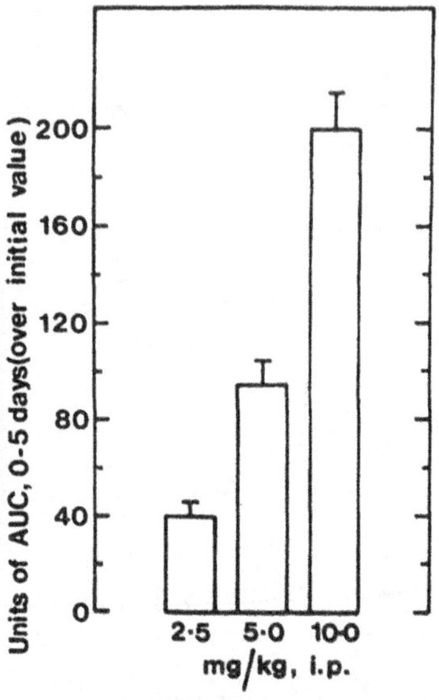

Fig. 9. Effect of forskolin on spontaneously hypertensive rats.

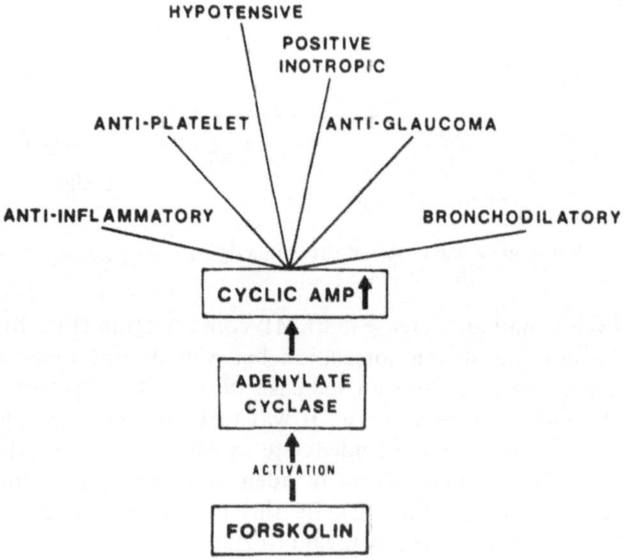

Fig. 10. Pharmacological properties of forskolin mediated by the activation of adenylate cyclase.

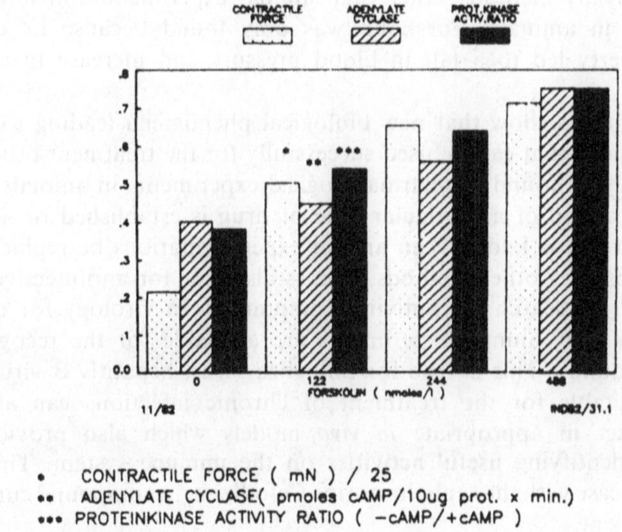

Fig. 11. Correlation between the contractile force in electrically stimulated left guinea-pig atria and the adenylate-cyclase activity and the degree of activation of the cAMP-dependent proteinkinase (Ca(++) = 1.025 mM).

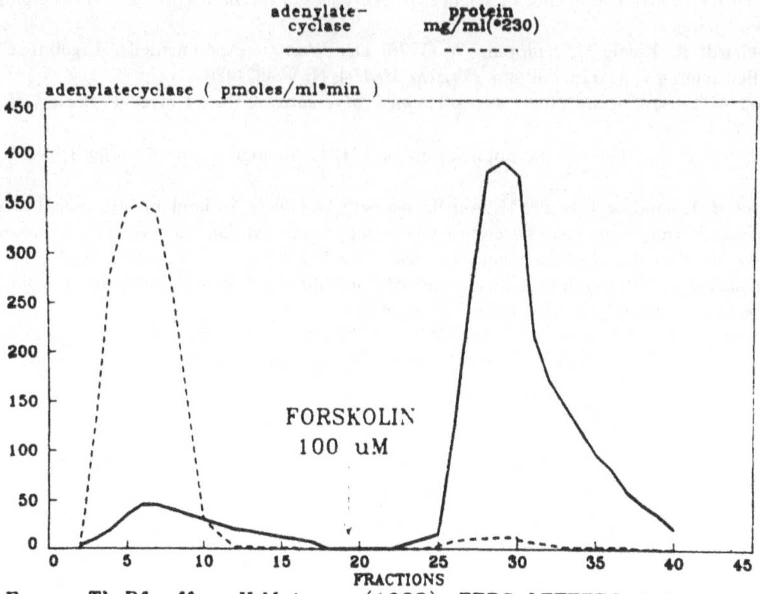

From: Th.Pfeuffer, H.Metzger (1982), FEBS LETTERS 146, 369–375

Fig. 12. Affinity chromatographic purification of solubilized rabbit myocardial adenylate cyclase on forskolin-sepharose.

be studied easily by methods other than animal experimentation have first to be detected in animals. Forskolin was only found because its cyclase activating property led to a fall in blood pressure and increase in cardiac contractility.

All these examples show that new biological phenomena leading to pharmacological actions that can be used successfully for the treatment of human diseases can only be found in pharmacological experiments in animals. Only if the mode of action of a particular type of drug is established or at least the site of its action is known, can animal experimentations be replaced for screening purposes by other methods. This is also true for antiinfectives and particularly for the search for antiviral compounds. In virology for certain types of viruses only animal experiments are available for the recognition of active compounds. This is true for influenza virus, hepatitis B virus, etc. Compounds suitable for the treatment of chronic infections can also be recognized better in appropriate *in vivo* models which also provide the possibility of identifying useful activities on the immune system. This was for example the case with the cephalosporine Cefodizime, a compound currently under development.

References

1. Jensen EV (1969) The science of science. In: *Advances in the Biosciences* 2: 5–17, Pergamon Press, Vieweg
2. Burkhardt R, Kienle G, Knipping W (1976) Der Wert tierexperimenteller Ergebnisse für die Beurteilung von Arzneimitteln. *Fortschr Med* 94, Nr 9: 482–486
3. Paton W (1984) *Man and mouse. Animals in medical research.* Oxford University Press, Oxford, New York
4. Sandow J (1986) Therapeutic applications of LHRH analogues. *The Releaser* 1, No 3: 3–8
5. Fraser HM, Sandow J, Seidel H, von Rechenberg W (1987) An implant of a gonadotropin releasing hormone agonist (buserelin) which suppresses ovarian function in the macaque for 3–5 months. *Acta Endocrinologica (Copenh)* 115: 521–527
6. Dohadwalla AN (1985) Biological activities of Forskolin. In: *Forskolin, its chemical, biological and medical potential,* Hoechst India Ltd. Bombay, 19–30
7. Metzger H (1985) Forskolin, an unique tool to study the properties and the regulation of adenylate cyclases. In: *Forskolin, its chemical, biological and medical potential,* Hoechst India Ltd., Bombay, 65–78

The manufacturer's authorised representative in the EU is Springer Nature Customer Service Centre GmbH, Europaplatz 3, 69115 Heidelberg, Germany. If you have any concerns regarding our products, please contact ProductSafety@springernature.com

Printed and bound by CPI Group (UK) Ltd, Croydon, CR0 4YY

30/09/2026

02225450-0015